MW00882194

The Top 100 Drug Interactions

A Guide to Patient Management

2016 Edition

Philip D. Hansten, PharmD
Professor Emeritus of Pharmacy
University of Washington
Seattle, Washington

John R. Horn, PharmD
Professor of Pharmacy
University of Washington
Seattle, Washington

Published by
H&H Publications, LLP, Box 1418
Freeland, WA 98249-1418 USA

Visit H&H Publications:
www.hanstenandhorn.com

Available from Amazon.com and other online stores
Printed by CreateSpace, an Amazon.com Company

i

Publisher's Note

This guide to drug interactions was prepared solely by the authors. It is not intended to replace more complete sources of drug interaction information.

The authors and publisher of this book have made every effort to ensure the accuracy of the information presented. Nevertheless, it is the responsibility of the reader to assess the appropriateness of the recommendations presented after consideration of patient specific factors and after consideration of any new developments in the field. The authors and publisher disclaim all responsibility for any errors or damage incurred as a consequence of the use of the information contained in this book.

Comments or suggestions? Visit our website at www.hanstenandhorn.com.

ISBN-13: 978-1522757139
ISBN-10: 1522757139

Table of Contents

Introduction

It is often difficult to distinguish clinically important from unimportant drug interactions. Given the lack of definitive epidemiological studies of drug interactions in patients, it is seldom possible to determine with certainty which interactions actually represent the most danger to public health. This book represents an attempt to identify drug interactions that should not be ignored in clinical practice. The original edition of this book contained about 100 interaction monographs. It has grown substantially and now contains over 8000 individual drug-drug interactions. The interactions are arranged according to *object drug* (the drug affected by the interaction) and *precipitant drug* (the drug causing the interaction). The precipitant drugs are grouped by mechanism (e.g., enzyme inhibitors or enzyme inducers) to show the types of interactions in which each object drug participates. Use the index to find drugs listed by their generic name. This book is intended to be a guide to drug interactions and the reader is reminded to check the cytochrome P450 table (see page vii) for additional drug combinations that may interact.

Information about the use of this book:
- This book employs an operational classification for drug interactions (see description of ORCA system on page VI).
- Note that the magnitude of drug interactions tends to vary widely (usually 6-8-fold or more) between patients and is usually difficult to predict. For that reason, we do not generally provide specific values defining the magnitude of an interaction. Even modest changes in the plasma concentration of drugs with narrow therapeutic ranges, or in patients with certain predisposing factors, can produce severe adverse effects.
- Some interactions, not yet reported in the literature, are included based on the known properties of the two drugs.
- Although it is often desirable to avoid adverse drug interactions by using non-interacting alternatives, few of the interactions in this book represent absolute contraindications. The prescriber is urged to carefully consider the risk-benefit ratio associated with the coadministration of interacting drugs.
- We have attempted to provide non-interacting alternatives for the object and/or precipitant drugs under the Comments or Management Class monograph headings. The prescriber should consider all patient variables before selecting an alternative agent. Drug product labeling should be consulted for full prescribing information.
- For the most part, this book does not include drug interactions with food, smoking, or drugs used primarily during surgery. Neither does it include predictable pharmacologic interactions such as additive CNS or bone marrow depression, renal toxins, or desirable drug-drug interactions.
- To obtain information on the mechanisms of drug interactions and access over 145 concise reviews of specific interactions and related topics, visit our website at www.hanstenandhorn.com.

New for the 2016 Edition
New monographs have been added and a number of current monographs have been revised. The CYP450 and transporter table has been updated with a number of new entries.

This is the seventeenth edition of The Top 100 Drug Interactions. We are gratified by the response to the book since the first edition was published in 2000. More than 300,000 copies of the various editions are in print, and it has been translated into Japanese, Korean, and French. We are pleased that several schools and colleges of pharmacy have adopted the book as a text for drug interaction and pharmaceutics courses. Substantial student discounts are available upon request. Several institutions have used our interaction classification approach as a basis for customizing their drug interaction alerting software. Suggestions and corrections are welcome at www.hanstenandhorn.com.

About the Authors:

Drs. Philip Hansten and John Horn are recognized as international authorities in the field of drug-drug interactions. Their combined experience exceeds 75 years of study in the field. Most of their scholarship has been on translational research designed to bring the basic principles of drug interactions into clinical focus. Combined, their drug interaction books have been translated into 7 languages and have sold more than one million copies worldwide since 1971. Hansten and Horn have lectured extensively in North America and in over two-dozen countries worldwide.

Operational Classification of Drug Interactions

The OpeRational ClassificAtion (ORCA) system for drug interactions used by Hansten and Horn in this book was developed by the Drug Interaction Foundation in an effort to improve the clinical utility of classification systems for drug interactions. (See reference below for more detailed description of ORCA.) As such, the classification system differs from all others in its fundamental approach to evaluation of potential interactions. The system assigns drug interactions to categories based on the *management* of the interaction (which is generally the primary issue confronting the health professional). The objective is to provide a classification system that practitioners will find both easier to use and of greater benefit as a clinical decision support tool than previous classification systems based on estimated "clinical significance" or levels of documentation. **Note: only drug interactions in Classes 1, 2, and 3 are included in this book.**

Class 1:	Avoid Combination (*Risk of combination outweighs benefit*)
Class 2:	Usually Avoid Combination (*Use only under special circumstances*) • Interactions for which there are clearly preferable alternatives for one or both drugs. • Interactions to avoid by using an alternative drug or other therapy unless the benefit is judged to outweigh the increased risk.
Class 3:	Minimize Risk (*Assess risk and take one or more of the following actions if needed*) • *Consider alternatives:* Alternatives may be available that are less likely to interact. • *Circumvent:* Take action to minimize the interaction (without avoiding combination). • *Monitor:* Early detection can minimize the risk of an adverse outcome.
Class 4:	No Special Precautions (*Risk of adverse outcome appears small*)
Class 5:	Ignore (*Evidence suggests that the drugs do not interact*)

Hansten PD, Horn JR, Hazlet TK. ORCA: OpeRational ClassificAtion of Drug Interactions. *J Am Pharm Assoc* 2001;41:161-5.

Cytochrome P450 Enzymes and Transporters Table

Inhibition or induction of cytochrome P450 (CYP450) drug metabolizing isozymes is a relatively common mechanism by which clinically important drug interactions occur. The recommended nomenclature for these enzymes is "CYP" to designate human cytochrome P450, followed by an Arabic number to designate the P450 family, followed by a capital letter to designate the subfamily; followed by an Arabic number to indicate the individual gene. Thus, examples of individual isozymes would include CYP1A2, CYP2C9, CYP2D6, etc. Entries on the table are supported by *in vivo* data. Some important characteristics of CYP450 isozymes include the following:

- Inhibition is substrate independent (e.g., a potent inhibitor of CYP3A4 is very likely to inhibit the metabolism of any drug metabolized by CYP3A4).
- Some (but **not** all) substrates are also inhibitors for the same enzyme, probably due to competitive inhibition of the enzyme (e.g., tacrine and CYP1A2 or verapamil and CYP3A4).
- Some inhibitors affect more than one enzyme or transporter (e.g., amiodarone inhibits CYP2C8, CYP2C9, CYP2D6, CYP3A4 and P-glycoprotein).
- The magnitude of inhibition of CYP450 enzymes tends to be dose related over the dosage range of the inhibitor (e.g., cimetidine 1200 mg/day is a more potent inhibitor than 400 mg/day).
- An inhibitor may produce inhibition of one isozyme at one dose, but require a larger dose of the inhibitor to inhibit another CYP isozyme (e.g., fluconazole inhibits CYP2C9 at low doses such as 100 mg/day, but significant inhibition of CYP3A4 requires larger doses such as 200-400 mg/day).
- Some substrates are metabolized by more than one isozyme (e.g., diazepam is metabolized by both CYP2C19 and CYP3A4, and tricyclic antidepressants are metabolized by many CYP450 isozymes).
- Most CYP450 isozyme inhibitors are themselves metabolized by the liver, but some are drugs with primarily renal elimination (e.g., cimetidine, fluconazole).
- Enantiomers may be metabolized by different isozymes. For example, the less potent anticoagulant R-warfarin is metabolized primarily by CYP1A2, while the more potent S-warfarin is metabolized primarily by CYP2C9. Thus, inhibitors of CYP1A2 tend to produce smaller increases in the hypoprothrombinemic response to warfarin, while CYP2C9 inhibitors can produce large increases in warfarin effect.

Drug transporters are also involved in many drug interactions. These transporters are found in many tissues, and they actively pump drug molecules either out of cells (efflux) or into cells (uptake). Many of the characteristics of CYP450 isozymes (above) apply to transporters as well. We have included P-glycoprotein (PGP), the organic anion transporter (OAT) and organic cation transporter (OCT) on the table.

Legend:

⊙ = Substrate for isozyme or transporter
↓ = Inhibitor (weak inhibitors = ↓)
↑ = Inducer (weak inducer = ↑)
* = Primary metabolic path for drugs with multiple pathways

Drug	1A2	2B6	2C8	2C9	2C19	2D6	3A4	PGP	OAT	OCT
Abiraterone (Zytiga)			↓			↓	⊙			
Acenocoumarol	⊙			⊙*	⊙					
Ado-trastuzumab (Kadcyla)							⊙			
Afatinib (Gilotrif)								⊙		
Alcohol (intoxication)[1]				↓						
Alfentanil (Alfenta)							⊙	⊙↓		
Alfuzosin (Uroxatral)							⊙			
Aliskiren (Tekturna)							⊙	⊙	⊙	
Almotriptan (Axert)						⊙	⊙			
Alosetron (Lotronex)	⊙			⊙			⊙			
Alprazolam (Xanax)							⊙			
Alprenolol						⊙				
Ambrisentan (Letairis)					⊙		⊙	⊙		
Amiodarone (Cordarone)			↓	↓		↓	⊙↓	↓		⊙
Aminoglutethimide	↑			↑			↑			
Amitriptyline (Elavil)	⊙				⊙	⊙*	⊙	⊙		
Amlodipine (Norvasc)							⊙	↓		
Amoxapine (Asendin)						⊙				
Amprenavir (Agenerase)					⊙		⊙*↓	⊙		
Anagrelide (Agrylin)	⊙									
Apixaban (Eliquis)							⊙	⊙		
Apremilast (Otezla)							⊙			
Aprepitant (Emend)	⊙			↑	⊙		⊙*↓			
Aripiprazole (Abilify)[2]						⊙*	⊙			
Armodafinil (Nuvigil)					↓		⊙↑			
Artemether (Coartem)		↑			↑		⊙↑			
Artemisinin	↓	⊙↑			⊙↑					
Asenapine (Saphris)	⊙					↓				
Astemizole							⊙			
Atazanavir (Reyataz)	↓						⊙↓	⊙		
Atenolol (Tenormin)										⊙
Axitinib (Inlyta)							⊙			
Atomoxetine (Strattera)						⊙				
Atorvastatin (Lipitor)							⊙	⊙↓	⊙↓	
Avanafil (Stendra)							⊙			
Axitinib (Inlyta)							⊙			
Azapropazone				⊙↓						
Azilsartan (Edarbi)				⊙						
Azithromycin (Zithromax)								⊙↓		
Barbiturates	↑			↑	↑		↑	↑		
Basiliximab (Simulect)							↓			
Bedaquiline (Sirturo)			⊙		⊙		⊙*			

Drug	1A2	2B6	2C8	2C9	2C19	2D6	3A4	PGP	OAT	OCT
Bendamustine (Treanda)	⊙									
Bepridil (Vascor)							⊙	↓		
Berberine (Goldenseal)				↓		↓	↓			
Betamethasone (Celestone)							⊙			
Bexarotene (Targretin)							⊙↑			
Bicalutamide (Casodex)							↓			
Boceprevir (Victrelis)							⊙↓	⊙		
Bortezomib (Velcade)	⊙				⊙		⊙*			
Bosentan (Tracleer)				⊙↑			⊙↑		⊙	
Bosutinib (Bosulif)							⊙			
Brentuximab (Adcetris)							⊙			
Brexpriprazole (Rexulti)						⊙	⊙			
Bromocriptine (Parlodel)							⊙			
Budesonide (Entocort)							⊙	⊙		
Bupivacaine (Sensorcaine)							⊙			
Buprenorphine (Subutex)							⊙			
Bupropion (Wellbutrin)		⊙				↓				
Buspirone (Buspar)							⊙			
Cabazitaxel (Jevtana)			⊙				⊙*			
Cabozantinib (Cometriq)							⊙			
Caffeine	⊙↓									
Canagliflozin (Invokana)								⊙↓		
Candesartan (Atacand)				⊙						
Capecitabine (Xeloda)				↓						
Carbamazepine (Tegretol)	↑	↑	⊙	↑	↑		⊙↑	↑		
Cariprazine (Vraylar)							⊙			
Carisoprodol (Soma)					⊙					
Carvedilol (Coreg)				⊙		⊙		⊙↓		
Celecoxib (Celebrex)				⊙		↓				
Ceritinib (Zykadia)				↓			⊙↓	⊙		
Cetirizine (Zyrtec)							⊙			
Cevimeline (Evoxac)						⊙	⊙			
Chloramphenicol					↓		↓			
Chloroquine (Aralen)			⊙				⊙↓			
Chlorpheniramine							⊙↓	⊙		
Chlorpromazine (Thorazine)	⊙						⊙↓			
Chlorpropamide (Diabinese)				⊙						
Cilostazol (Pletal)					⊙		⊙↓			
Cimetidine (Tagamet)	↓				↓	↓			↓	⊙↓
Cinacalcet (Sensipar)	⊙					⊙↓	⊙			
Ciprofloxacin (Cipro)	↓						↓			
Cisapride (Propulsid)							⊙			
Citalopram (Celexa)					⊙*	⊙↓	⊙	⊙		
Clarithromycin (Biaxin)							⊙↓	↓	↓	
Clobazam (Onfi)		⊙			⊙	↓	⊙*↑			
Clomipramine (Anafranil)	⊙				⊙	⊙*	⊙			
Clonazepam (Klonopin)			⊙				⊙			

Drug	1A2	2B6	2C8	2C9	2C19	2D6	3A4	PGP	OAT	OCT
Clonidine (Catapres)						⊙				
Clopidogrel (Plavix)	⊙	↓	↓	⊙	⊙*↓		⊙	⊙		
Clozapine (Clozaril)³	⊙*				⊙	⊙	⊙			
Cobicistat (Stribild)						↓	⊙↓	↓	↓	
Cobimetinib (Cotellic)							⊙	⊙		
Codeine						⊙				
Colchicine (Colcrys)							⊙	⊙		
Conivaptan (Vaprisol)							⊙↓	↓		
Co-trimoxazole (Septra)				↓	⊙↓		⊙			
Crizotinib (Xalkori)							⊙↓			
Cyclobenzaprine (Flexeril)	⊙						⊙			
Cyclophosphamide (Cytoxan)		⊙*↓					⊙			
Cyclosporine (Neoral)							⊙↓	⊙↓	↓	
Dabigatran (Pradaxa)								⊙		
Dabrafenib (Tafinlar)			⊙	↑			⊙↑	⊙		
Daclatasvir (Daklinza)							⊙	↓	↓	
Dalfopristin (Synercid)							↓			
Danazol (Danocrine)							↓			
Dapsone (Avlosulfon)							⊙			
Darifenacin (Enablex)						⊙↓	⊙			
Darunavir (Prezista)							⊙↓			
Dasabuvir (Viekira Pak)			⊙					⊙		
Dasatinib (Sprycel)							⊙↓	⊙		
Daunorubicin (Cerubidine)							⊙			
Debrisoquin						⊙				
Deferasirox (Exjade)	⊙		↓				↑			
Delavirdine (Rescriptor)				↓	↓		⊙↓			
Desipramine (Norpramin)						⊙	⊙*			
Desloratadine (Clarinex)							⊙			
Desvenlafaxine (Pristiq)						↓	⊙			
Dexamethasone (Decadron)							⊙↑	⊙↑		
Dexlansoprazole (Kapidex)					⊙		⊙			
Dextromethorphan						⊙*	⊙			
Diazepam (Valium)					⊙*		⊙			
Diclofenac (Voltaren)			⊙	⊙			⊙			
Digoxin (Lanoxin)								⊙		
Dihydrocodeine						⊙				
Dihydroergotamine							⊙			
Diltiazem (Cardizem)							⊙↓	⊙↓		
Diphenhydramine (Benadryl)	⊙				⊙	⊙*↓				
Disopyramide (Norpace)							⊙			↓
Disulfiram (Antabuse)				↓			⊙			
Docetaxel (Taxotere)							⊙	⊙		
Dofetilide (Tikosyn)										⊙
Dolasetron (Anzemet)						⊙*	⊙			

x

Drug	1A2	2B6	2C8	2C9	2C19	2D6	3A4	PGP	OAT	OCT
Dolutegravir (Tivicay)										↓
Domperidone						⊙	⊙			
Donepezil (Aricept)						⊙	⊙*			
Doxepin (Sinequan)				⊙	⊙	⊙*				
Doxorubicin (Adriamycin)							⊙	⊙		
Doxifluridine				↓						
Dronabinol (Marinol)				⊙						
Dronedarone (Multaq)						↓	⊙↓	↓		
Droperidol (Inapsine)							⊙	⊙		
Duloxetine (Cymbalta)	⊙*					⊙↓		↓		
Dutasteride (Avodart)							⊙			
Ebastine (Kestine)							⊙			
Edoxaban (Savaysa)								⊙		
Efavirenz (Sustiva)		⊙*↑		↓	↑		⊙↑			
Eletriptan (Relpax)							⊙	⊙		
Eliglustat (Cerdelga)						⊙*↓	⊙	⊙↓		
Eltrombopag (Promacta)									↓	
Eluxadoline (Viberzi)									⊙	
Elvitegravir (Stribild)							⊙			
Encainide						⊙				
Enoxacin (Penetrex)	↓									
Enzalutamide (Xtandi)			⊙*	↑	↑		⊙↑			
Eplerenone (Inspra)							⊙			
Ergotamine (Ergomar)							⊙			
Erlotinib (Tarceva)	⊙		⊙				⊙*	⊙↓		
Erythromycin (E-Mycin)							⊙↓	⊙↓	↓	
Escitalopram (Lexapro)					⊙*	⊙↓	⊙			
Eslicarbazepine (Aptiom)					↓		↑			
Esomeprazole (Nexium)					⊙*↓		⊙			
Estazolam (Prosom)							⊙			
Eszopiclone (Lunesta)							⊙			
Ethinyl Estradiol	↓						⊙↓	⊙		
Ethosuximide (Zarontin)							⊙			
Etoposide (Vepesid)							⊙	⊙		
Etravirine (Intelence)				⊙↓	⊙*↓		⊙↑			
Everolimus (Afinitor)							⊙	⊙		
Exemestane (Aromasin)							⊙			
Felbamate (Felbatol)					↓					
Felodipine (Plendil)							⊙			
Fenofibrate (Tricor)								↓		
Fentanyl (Sublimaze)							⊙	⊙		
Fesoterodine (Toviaz)						⊙	⊙*			
Fexofenadine (Allegra)								⊙	⊙	
Fidaxomicin (Dificid)								⊙		
Finasteride (Proscar)							⊙			
Fingolimod (Gilenya)						⊙	⊙			
Flecainide (Tambocor)	⊙					⊙*↓				

Drug	1A2	2B6	2C8	2C9	2C19	2D6	3A4	PGP	OAT	OCT
Flibanserin (Addyi)					⊙		⊙*	↓		
Fluconazole (Diflucan)[4]				↓	↓		↓			
Fluorouracil (5-FU)				↓						
Fluoxetine (Prozac)[5]				⊙↓	⊙↓	⊙*↓	↓			
Flurazepam (Dalmane)							⊙			
Flurbiprofen (Ansaid)				⊙						
Flutamide (Eulexin)	⊙									
Fluticasone (Flonase)							⊙			
Fluvastatin (Lescol)			⊙	⊙↓					⊙	
Fluvoxamine (Luvox)	⊙↓			↓	↓	⊙*↓	↓			
Fosamprenavir (Lexiva)							⊙↓			
Frovatriptan (Frova)	⊙									
Galantamine (Reminyl)						⊙↓	⊙*			
Gefitinib (Iressa)						⊙	⊙	⊙		
Gemfibrozil (Lopid)			⊙↓	↓					↓	
Glimepiride (Amaryl)				⊙						
Glipizide (Glucotrol)				⊙						
Glyburide (DiaBeta)				⊙				⊙		
Granisetron (Kytril)							⊙			
Grapefruit[6]							↓	↓	↓	
Griseofulvin (Grisactin)				↑			↑			
Guanfacine (Intuniv)							⊙			
Halofantrine (Halfan)						↓	⊙			
Haloperidol (Haldol)						⊙*↓	⊙			
Hydrocodone (Vicodin)						⊙	⊙*			
Hydroxychloroquine						↓				
Ibrutinib (Imbruvica)						⊙	⊙*			
Ibuprofen (Advil, Motrin)			⊙	⊙						
Idelalisib (Zydelig)							⊙↓			
Ifosfamide (Ifex)		⊙					⊙			
Iloperidone (Fanapt)						⊙	⊙			
Imatinib (Gleevec)			⊙	↓		↓	⊙↓	⊙		
Imipramine (Tofranil)	⊙				⊙	⊙*	⊙			
Indacaterol (Arcapta)							⊙	⊙		
Indinavir (Crixivan)							⊙↓	⊙↓		
Indiplon	⊙						⊙			
Indomethacin (Indocin)				⊙						
Interleukin-10							↓			
Irbesartan (Avapro)				⊙						
Irinotecan (Camptosar)							⊙	⊙		
Isavuconazonium (Cresemba)		↑					⊙↓	↓		
Isoniazid (INH, Nydrazid)					↓		↓			
Isradipine (DynaCirc)							⊙			
Itraconazole (Sporanox)							⊙↓	⊙↓		
Ivabradine (Corlanor)							⊙			
Ivacaftor (Kalydeco)							⊙↓	↓		

Drug	1A2	2B6	2C8	2C9	2C19	2D6	3A4	PGP	OAT	OCT
Ixabepilone (Ixempra)							⊙			
Ixazomib (Ninlaro)							⊙			
Ketamine (Ketalar)		⊙		⊙			⊙			
Ketoconazole (Nizoral)							⊙↓	↓		
Labetalol (Normodyne)						⊙				
Lacosamide (Vimpat)					⊙					
Lansoprazole (Prevacid)					⊙		⊙			↓
Lapatinib (Tykerb)			⊙↓		⊙		⊙*↓	⊙↓		
Ledipasvir (Harvoni)								⊙↓		
Leflunomide (Arava)	⊙			↓	⊙					
Lenvatinib (Lenvima)							⊙	⊙		
Letrozole (Femara)							⊙			
Levofloxacin (Levaquin)										↓
Levomethadyl (Orlaam)							⊙			
Levomilnacipran (Fetzima)							⊙			
Lidocaine	⊙*						⊙			
Linagliptin (Tradjenta)							↓	⊙	⊙	
Lomitapide (Juxtapid)							⊙↓	↓		
Loperamide (Imodium)			⊙				⊙	⊙		
Lopinavir (Kaletra)							⊙			
Loratadine (Claritin)						⊙	⊙*	⊙		
Lorcaserin (Belviq)						↓				
Losartan (Cozaar)[7]				⊙*			⊙			
Lovastatin (Mevacor)							⊙*	⊙↓	⊙	
Loxapine (Loxitane)	⊙*					⊙	⊙			
Lumacaftor (Orkambi)							↑			
Lumefantrine (Coartem)						↓	⊙			
Lurasidone (Latuda)							⊙			
Macitentan (Opsumit)					⊙		⊙*			
Maprotiline (Ludiomil)						⊙				
Maraviroc (Selzentry)							⊙	⊙		
Mefloquine (Lariam)							⊙	⊙↓		
Melatonin	⊙*			⊙						
Meloxicam (Mobic)				⊙*			⊙			
Mephenytoin (Mesantoin)					⊙					
Meropenem (Merrem)									⊙	
Mesoridazine (Serentil)						⊙				
Metformin (Glucophage)										⊙
Methadone		⊙*			⊙	⊙↓	⊙			
Methamphetamine						⊙				
Methotrexate									⊙	
Methylprednisolone							⊙	⊙		
Metoclopramide (Reglan)						⊙				
Metoprolol (Lopressor)						⊙				
Metronidazole (Flagyl)				↓						
Mexiletine (Mexitil)	⊙↓					⊙*				
Mianserin						⊙				

xiii

Drug	1A2	2B6	2C8	2C9	2C19	2D6	3A4	PGP	OAT	OCT
Miconazole (Monistat)				↓			↓			
Midazolam (Versed)							⊙			
Mifepristone (Korlym)		↓		↓			⊙↓	↓		
Mirabegron (Myrbetriq)						⊙↓	⊙*	⊙		⊙
Mirtazapine (Remeron)	⊙					⊙	⊙			
Mitomycin							⊙			
Mitotane (Lysodren)							↑			
Moclobemide (Manerix)					⊙↓	↓				
Modafinil (Provigil)[8]				↓	↓		⊙↑			
Mometasone (Nasonex)							⊙			
Montelukast (Singulair)			⊙*	⊙			⊙		⊙	
Morphine							⊙			⊙
Nadolol (Corgard)							⊙			
Nafcillin (Unipen)				↑?			↑			
Naloxegol (Movantik)							⊙	⊙		
Naproxen (Naprosyn)				⊙						
Nefazodone							⊙↓			
Nateglinide (Starlix)				⊙*			⊙			
Nebivolol (Bystolic)						⊙				
Nelfinavir (Viracept)[9]				↑	⊙		⊙↓	⊙↓		
Netupitant (Akynzeo)				⊙		⊙	⊙*↓			
Nevirapine (Viramune)		⊙					⊙↑			
Nicardipine (Cardene)							⊙↓	↓		
Nifedipine (Adalat)							⊙	↓		
Nilotinib (Tasigna)							⊙↓	⊙		
Nimodipine (Nimotop)							⊙			
Nintedanib (Ofev)							⊙	⊙		
Nisoldipine (Sular)							⊙			
Nitrendipine (Baypress)							⊙			
Norfloxacin (Norflox)	↓									
Nortriptyline (Pamelor)						⊙*	⊙	⊙		
Olanzapine (Zyprexa)	⊙*					⊙				
Olaparib (Lynparza)							⊙			
Ombitasvir (Technivie)								⊙		
Omeprazole (Prilosec)					⊙*↓		⊙			
Ondansetron (Zofran)	⊙*					⊙	⊙	⊙		
Oritavancin (Orbactiv)				↓			↑			
Oseltamivir (Tamiflu)								⊙		
Osimertinib (Tagrisso)							⊙			
Ospemifene (Osphena)				⊙	⊙		⊙*			
Oxcarbazepine (Trileptal)					↓		↑			
Oxybutynin (Ditropan)							⊙			
Oxycodone (Percodan)						⊙	⊙*			
Paclitaxel (Taxol)			⊙				⊙	⊙		
Palbociclib (Ibrance)							⊙			
Paliperidone (Invega)						⊙		⊙		
Palonosetron (Aloxi)	⊙					⊙*	⊙			

Drug	1A2	2B6	2C8	2C9	2C19	2D6	3A4	PGP	OAT	OCT
Panobinostat (Farydak)				⊙		⊙↓	⊙*			
Pantoprazole (Protonix)					⊙*		⊙			
Paricalcitol (Zemplar)							⊙			
Paritaprevir (Technivie)						⊙*	⊙↓	⊙↓		
Paroxetine (Paxil)						⊙↓	⊙			
Pazopanib (Votrient)						↓	⊙↓			
Pentamidine (Pentam)					⊙					
Perampanel (Fycompa)							⊙			
Perhexiline (Pexid)						⊙				
Perphenazine (Trilafon)						⊙↓				
Phenobarbital	↑	↑		⊙↑	⊙↑		↑			
Phenytoin (Dilantin)	↑	↑	⊙	⊙*↑	⊙↑		↑	↑		
Pimozide (Orap)	⊙					⊙	⊙*			
Pioglitazone (Actos)[17]			⊙*	⊙			⊙			
Pirfenidone (Esbriet)	⊙									
Piroxicam (Feldene)				⊙						
Pitavastatin (Livalo)				⊙					⊙	
Plicamycin (Mithracin)							⊙			
Pomalidomide (Pomalyst)	⊙*						⊙	⊙		
Ponatinib (Iclusig)			⊙			⊙	⊙	↓		
Posaconazole (Noxafil)							↓	⊙↓		
Prasugrel (Effient)		⊙		⊙	⊙		⊙			
Pravastatin (Pravachol)									⊙	
Praziquantel (Biltricide)							⊙			
Prednisolone							⊙			
Prednisone							⊙	⊙		
Primidone (Mysoline)	↑			↑	↑		↑			
Probenecid (Benemid)									⊙↓	
Procainamide (Procan)[15]										⊙
Proguanil[15]					⊙					
Promethazine (Phenergan)						⊙↓				
Propafenone (Rythmol)	⊙					⊙*↓	⊙	↓		
Propofol (Diprivan)		⊙								
Propoxyphene (Darvon)						⊙↓	⊙*↓			
Propranolol (Inderal)	⊙					⊙	⊙*			
Protriptyline (Vivactil)						⊙				
Quazepam (Doral)							⊙			
Quetiapine (Seroquel)						⊙	⊙*			
Quinacrine						↓	⊙			
Quinidine (Quinidex)						↓	⊙	⊙↓		⊙↓
Quinine						↓	⊙	↓		
Quinupristin (Synercid)							↓			
Rabeprazole (Aciphex)					⊙					
Raltegravir (Isentress)								⊙		
Ramelteon (Rozerem)	⊙*			⊙			⊙			
Ranolazine (Ranexa)						⊙↓	⊙*↓	⊙↓		
Rasagiline (Azilect)	⊙									

Drug	1A2	2B6	2C8	2C9	2C19	2D6	3A4	PGP	OAT	OCT
Regorafenib (Stivarga)							⊙			
Repaglinide (Prandin)			⊙				⊙		⊙	
Rifabutin (Mycobutin)							⊙↑			
Rifaximin (Xifaxan)[18]							⊙	⊙		
Rifampin (Rimactane)	↑	↑	↑	↑	↑		↑	⊙↑	↓	↑
Rifapentine (Priftin)						↑	↑			
Rilpivirine (Edurant)							⊙			
Riluzole (Rilutek)	⊙									
Riociguat (Adempas)[16]			⊙				⊙	⊙		
Risperidone (Risperdal)						⊙*↓	⊙	⊙		
Ritonavir (Norvir)[10]		↑			↑	↓	⊙↓	⊙↓		
Rivaroxaban (Xarelto)							⊙	⊙		
Roflumilast (Daliresp)	⊙						⊙			
Rolapitant (Varubi)						↓	⊙	↓		
Romidepsin (Istodax)							⊙	⊙		
Ropinirole (Requip)	⊙									
Ropivacaine (Naropin)	⊙*						⊙			
Rosiglitazone (Avandia)			⊙*	⊙						
Rosuvastatin (Crestor)				⊙						⊙
Rufinamide (Banzel)							↑			
Ruxolitinib (Jakafi)							⊙			
Salmeterol (Serevent)							⊙			
Saquinavir (Invirase)							⊙↓	⊙↓		
Saxagliptin (Onglyza)							⊙	⊙		
Secobarbital	↑				↑					
Selegiline (Eldepryl)	⊙	⊙					⊙			
Sertindole (Serlect)						⊙	⊙			
Sertraline (Zoloft)					⊙*	⊙↓	⊙	⊙		
Sildenafil (Viagra)				⊙			⊙*			
Silodosin (Rapaflo)							⊙	⊙		
Simeprevir (Olysio)	↓						⊙*↓	⊙↓	⊙↓	
Simvastatin (Zocor)						⊙	⊙*			⊙
Sirolimus (Rapammune)							⊙	⊙		
Sitagliptin (Januvia)							⊙	⊙	⊙	
Smoking	↑									
Sofosbuvir (Sovaldi)								⊙		
Solifenacin (Vesicare)							⊙			
Sonidegib (Odomzo)							⊙			
Sorafenib (Nexavar)							⊙	⊙		
St. John's wort[11]		↑		↑	↑		↑	↑		
Sufentanil (Sufenta)							⊙			
Sulfamethizole				↓						
Sulfamethoxazole (Bactrim)				⊙*↓			⊙			
Sulfaphenazole				↓						
Sulfinpyrazone (Anturane)				↓						
Sunitinib (Sutent)							⊙	⊙↓		
Suvorexant (Belsomra)							⊙↓			

xvi

Drug	1A2	2B6	2C8	2C9	2C19	2D6	3A4	PGP	OAT	OCT
Tacrine (Cognex)	⊙↓									
Tacrolimus (Prograf)							⊙	⊙↓		
Tadalafil (Cialis)							⊙			
Tamoxifen (Nolvadex)[12]				↓		⊙	⊙*↓	↓		
Tamsulosin (Flomax)						⊙	⊙			
Tasimelteon (Hetlioz)	⊙						⊙			
Telaprevir (Incivek)							⊙↓	⊙↓		
Telithromycin (Ketek)							⊙↓	↓		
Temsirolimus (Torisel)							⊙	⊙		
Teniposide (Vumon)							⊙	⊙		
Terbinafine (Lamisil)						↓				
Terfenadine							⊙	⊙		
Testosterone							⊙			
Tetrabenazine (Xenazine)						⊙				
Tetrahydrocannabinol				⊙*			⊙			
Thalidomide (Thalomid)					⊙					
Theophylline	⊙*						⊙			
Thiabendazole (Mintezol)	⊙↓									
Thioridazine (Mellaril)	⊙					⊙*↓	⊙			
Tiagabine (Gabitril)							⊙			
Ticagrelor (Brilinta)							⊙↓	↓		
Ticlopidine (Ticlid)	↓	↓			↓					
Timolol (Blocadren)						⊙				
Tinidazole (Tindamax)							⊙			
Tipranavir (Aptivus)							⊙	⊙↑	↓	
Tizanidine (Zanaflex)	⊙									
Tofacitinib (Xeljanz)							⊙			
Tolbutamide (Orinase)				⊙						
Tolterodine (Detrol)						⊙*	⊙			
Tolvaptan (Samsca)							⊙	⊙↓		
Topiramate (Topamax)					↓		⊙↑			
Toremifene (Fareston)						↓	⊙			
Torsemide (Demadex)				⊙						
Trabectedin (Yondelis)							⊙	⊙		
Tramadol (Ultram)		⊙				⊙*	⊙			
Trazodone (Desyrel)						⊙*	⊙			
Treprostinil (Tyvaso)			⊙							
Triamcinolone (Aristocort)							⊙			
Triamterene (Dyrenium)	⊙*						⊙			
Triazolam (Halcion)							⊙			
Trimethoprim (Septra)		↓								↓
Trimipramine (Surmontil)						⊙				
Troglitazone (Rezulin)							↑			
Troleandomycin (TAO)							↓			
Uliprista (Ella)							⊙			
Umeclidinium (Incruse Ellipta)								⊙		

Drug	1A2	2B6	2C8	2C9	2C19	2D6	3A4	PGP	OAT	OCT
Valdecoxib (Bextra)				⊙			⊙			
Valproic Acid (Depakote)				↓						
Valsartan (Diovan)				⊙						
Vandetanib (Caprelsa)							⊙			
Vardenafil (Levitra)							⊙			
Vemurafenib (Zelboraf)	↓					↓	⊙↑			
Venlafaxine (Effexor)					⊙	⊙*↓	⊙	⊙		
Verapamil (Calan)[14]							⊙↓	⊙↓		⊙↓
Vesnarinone							⊙			
Vilanterol (Breo Ellipta)							⊙	⊙		
Vilazodone (Viibryd)					⊙	⊙	⊙*			
Vinblastine (Velban)							⊙↑	⊙		
Vincristine (Oncovin)							⊙	⊙		
Vinorelbine (Navelbine)							⊙	⊙		
Vismodegib (Erivedge)							⊙			
Vorapaxar (Zontivity)							⊙			
Voriconazole (Vfend)				⊙↓	⊙↓		⊙↓			
Vortioxetine (Brintellix)				⊙	⊙	⊙*	⊙			
R-Warfarin (Coumadin)	⊙*				⊙		⊙			
S-Warfarin (Coumadin)				⊙*			⊙			
Yohimbine						⊙	⊙			
Zafirlukast (Accolate)				⊙*↓			⊙↓			
Zaleplon (Sonata)							⊙			
Zileuton (Zyflo)	⊙↓									
Ziprasidone (Geodon)[13]							⊙			
Zolmitriptan (Zolmig)	⊙									
Zolpidem (Ambien)	⊙			⊙			⊙*			
Zonisamide (Zonegran)						⊙	⊙			
Zopiclone (Imovane)			⊙				⊙			

Footnotes for Cytochrome P450 Enzymes & Transporters Table

1. Chronic alcohol abuse can result in increased CYP2C9 activity.
2. Aripiprazole is metabolized to an active metabolite, dehydroaripiprazole.
3. The role of CYP3A4 in clozapine metabolism is controversial. Clozapine does not appear to interact with itraconazole or grapefruit juice.
4. Fluconazole inhibition of CYP3A4 is dose related; 100 mg/day usually has little effect, but CYP3A4 inhibition occurs at 200 to 400 mg/day or more, depending on the substrate.
5. Fluoxetine's major metabolite (norfluoxetine) has a very long half-life and is also a potent inhibitor of CYP2D6; thus, CYP2D6 inhibition may persist for several weeks after stopping fluoxetine.
6. The inhibitory effect of grapefruit juice (GFJ) on CYP3A4 is dose related. A single glass of GFJ produces modest CYP3A4 inhibition while multiple glasses daily for several days can produce marked inhibition of CYP3A4. GFJ appears to affect only gut wall CYP3A4, but some effect on hepatic CYP3A4 has not been ruled out.
7. CYP2C9 converts losartan to an active metabolite.
8. Induction of CYP3A4 by modafinil appears to be more intestinal than hepatic.
9. Nelfinavir has been reported to decrease serum concentrations of methadone and ethinyl estradiol, suggesting that it might act as a CYP3A4 inducer in some situations.
10. Long-term ritonavir can *induce* CYP3A4 and possibly CYP1A2, CYP2C9, and P-glycoprotein. Ritonavir may induce CYP2B6 more rapidly.

11. St. John's wort may also induce other CYP450 isozymes such as CYP2C9, but more clinical data are needed. Single dose St. John's wort may inhibit P-glycoprotein.
12. Tamoxifen is predominantly metabolized by CYP3A4 to inactive metabolites, but CYP2D6 is responsible for converting tamoxifen to active metabolites.
13. About one-third of ziprasidone is metabolized by CYP3A4 and about two-thirds are metabolized by aldehyde oxidase.
14. Verapamil may induce P-glycoprotein during chronic administration.
15. CYP2C19 converts proguanil to an active metabolite.
16. CYP1A1 is primary pathway of metabolism.
17. Pioglitazone is metabolized by CYP2C8 to 2 active metabolites.
18. Rifaximin is minimally absorbed from the GI tract, but cyclosporine (inhibitor of both P-glycoprotein and CYP3A4) increased rifaximin AUC by 124-fold.

OBJECT DRUGS		PRECIPITANT DRUGS
ACE Inhibitors (ACEI):		Tizanidine (Zanaflex)
Benazepril (Lotensin)	Moexipril (Univasc)	
Captopril (Capoten)	Perindopril (Aceon)	
Enalapril (Vasotec)	Quinapril (Accupril)	
Fosinopril (Monopril)	Ramipril (Altace)	
Lisinopril (Prinivil)	Trandolapril (Mavik)	

COMMENTS: Patients on ACEI have developed severe hypotension after starting tizanidine therapy. Tizanidine, like the antihypertensive drug clonidine, is an alpha-2 adrenergic agonist, and may have additive hypotensive effects with ACE inhibitors.

CLASS 3: ASSESS RISK & TAKE ACTION IF NECESSARY
* *Consider Alternative*: In patients taking ACEI, consider using muscle relaxants other than tizanidine (that are not alpha-2 adrenergic agonists). Some other muscle relaxants can also cause hypotension, but the risk is probably less than for tizanidine.
* *Monitor*: If tizanidine is used in a patient taking an ACEI, monitor cardiovascular status carefully for evidence of an acute hypotensive reaction.

OBJECT DRUGS	PRECIPITANT DRUGS	
Acetaminophen	**Enzyme Inducers:**	
(Tylenol)	Barbiturates	Phenytoin (Dilantin)
	Carbamazepine (Tegretol)	Primidone (Mysoline)
	Efavirenz (Sustiva)	Rifabutin (Mycobutin)
	Isoniazid (INH)	Rifampin (Rifadin)
	Nevirapine (Viramune)	Rifapentine (Priftin)
	Oxcarbazepine (Trileptal)	St. John's wort

COMMENTS: Enzyme inducers have been reported to increase the formation of a toxic acetaminophen metabolite, thus increasing the risk of hepatotoxicity in patients taking overdoses of acetaminophen (or large and/or prolonged therapeutic doses). The analgesic effect of acetaminophen may also be reduced by enzyme inducers due to enhanced acetaminophen metabolism. Isoniazid has a biphasic effect, first reducing and then increasing the formation of toxic acetaminophen metabolites.

MANAGEMENT CLASS 3: ASSESS RISK & TAKE ACTION IF NECESSARY
* *Circumvent/Minimize*: Patients on enzyme inducers should avoid prolonged use of large therapeutic doses of acetaminophen. A safe amount of acetaminophen for such patients is not established, but it would be prudent to limit intake of acetaminophen to 2 g/day or less.
* *Consider Alternative*: Since acetaminophen analgesia may be reduced; doses considered safe may be ineffective. Thus, it may be necessary to use alternative analgesics. Note, however, that salicylates and NSAIDs may produce additive toxicity with excessive alcohol intake.

OBJECT DRUGS	PRECIPITANT DRUGS	
Alfuzosin (Uroxatral)	**Antimicrobials:**	
	Ciprofloxacin (Cipro)	Posaconazole (Noxafil)
	Clarithromycin (Biaxin)	Quinupristin (Synercid)
	Erythromycin (E-Mycin)	Telithromycin (Ketek)
	Fluconazole (Diflucan)	Troleandomycin (TAO)
	Itraconazole (Sporanox)	Voriconazole (Vfend)
	Ketoconazole (Nizoral)	

COMMENTS: Alfuzosin is primarily metabolized by CYP3A4, and these antimicrobial agents are inhibitors of CYP3A4. Based on a more than 3-fold increase in alfuzosin AUC with ketoconazole, the alfuzosin labeling states that combined use of alfuzosin with potent CYP3A4 inhibitors is contraindicated. Although not all of these antimicrobials have equal potency as CYP3A4 inhibitors, they all would be expected to produce substantial increases in alfuzosin plasma concentrations.

CLASS 2: USE ONLY IF BENEFIT FELT TO OUTWEIGH RISK
* *Use Alternative*:
  Azole Antifungals: Fluconazole appears to be a less potent inhibitor of CYP3A4 than itraconazole or ketoconazole, but in larger doses it also inhibits CYP3A4. **Terbinafine** (Lamisil) does not appear to affect CYP3A4.
  Macrolide Antibiotics: Unlike erythromycin, clarithromycin and troleandomycin, other macrolides such as **azithromycin** (Zithromax) and **dirithromycin*** do not appear to inhibit CYP3A4. (*not available in US)

1

<u>Telithromycin</u>: The use of **azithromycin** (Zithromax) or a quinolone antibiotic other than ciprofloxacin should be considered.
- *Monitor*: If alfuzosin is used with a CYP3A4 inhibitor, monitor blood pressure for evidence of hypotension. Placing the patient in the supine position or additional measures (intravenous fluids, vasopressors) may be necessary if hypotension occurs.

OBJECT DRUGS	PRECIPITANT DRUGS	
Alfuzosin (Uroxatral)	**Enzyme Inhibitors:**	
	Amiodarone (Cordarone)	**Diltiazem** (Cardizem)
	Amprenavir (Agenerase)	**Dronedarone** (Multaq)
	Aprepitant (Emend)	**Grapefruit**
	Atazanavir (Reyataz)	**Indinavir** (Crixivan)
	Boceprevir (Victrelis)	**Lomitapide** (Juxtapid)
	Ceritinib (Zykadia)	**Mifepristone** (Korlym)
	Cobicistat (Stribild)	**Nelfinavir** (Viracept)
	Conivaptan (Vaprisol)	**Ritonavir** (Norvir)
	Cyclosporine (Neoral)	**Saquinavir** (Invirase)
	Darunavir (Prezista)	**Telaprevir** (Incivek)
	Delavirdine (Rescriptor)	**Verapamil** (Isoptin)

COMMENTS: Alfuzosin is primarily metabolized by CYP3A4, and these agents are inhibitors of CYP3A4. The alfuzosin labeling states that combined use of alfuzosin with potent CYP3A4 inhibitors is contraindicated. Although not all of these drugs have equal potency as CYP3A4 inhibitors, they all would be expected to produce substantial increases in alfuzosin plasma concentrations.

CLASS 2: USE ONLY IF BENEFIT FELT TO OUTWEIGH RISK
- *Use Alternative*:
  Calcium Channel Blockers: Calcium channel blockers other than diltiazem and verapamil are unlikely to significantly inhibit the metabolism of alfuzosin.
  Grapefruit: Orange juice does not appear to inhibit CYP3A4.
- *Monitor*: If alfuzosin is used with a CYP3A4 inhibitor, monitor blood pressure for evidence of hypotension. Placing the patient in the supine position or additional measures (intravenous fluids, vasopressors) may be necessary if hypotension occurs.

OBJECT DRUGS	PRECIPITANT DRUGS	
Aliskiren (Tekturna)	**Angiotensin Receptor Blockers:**	
	Azilsartan (Edarbi)	**Losartan** (Cozaar)
	Candesartan (Atacand)	**Olmesartan** (Benicar)
	Eprosartan (Teveten)	**Telmisartan** (Micardis)
	Irbesartan (Avapro)	**Valsartan** (Diovan)

COMMENTS: Concurrent use of renin inhibitors and angiotensin receptor blockers (ARBs) may lead to additive hyperkalemic and hypotensive effects, especially in the presence of one or more predisposing factors such as significant renal impairment, severe diabetes, potassium supplements, high potassium diet, and advanced age. Other drugs that may exhibit hyperkalemic activity include **ACE inhibitors, drospirenone** (Yasmin), **heparins, nonselective beta-blockers, NSAIDs, COX-2 inhibitors, cyclosporine, tacrolimus, succinylcholine, pentamidine, trimethoprim,** and **potassium-containing salt substitutes**. The product information states that aliskiren is contraindicated in patients with diabetes who are receiving ARBs.

CLASS 3: ASSESS RISK & TAKE ACTION IF NECESSARY
- *Monitor*: Monitor serum potassium concentrations and blood pressure, especially in patients with predisposing factors such as renal disease, diabetes, and advanced age.

OBJECT DRUGS	PRECIPITANT DRUGS	
Aliskiren (Tekturna)	**ACE inhibitors:**	
	Benazepril (Lotensin)	**Moexipril** (Univasc)
	Captopril (Capoten)	**Perindopril** (Aceon)
	Enalapril (Vasotec)	**Quinapril** (Accupril)
	Fosinopril (Monopril)	**Ramipril** (Altace)
	Lisinopril (Prinivil)	**Trandolapril** (Mavik)

COMMENTS: Concurrent use of renin inhibitors and angiotensin converting enzyme inhibitors (ACEI) may lead to additive hyperkalemic and hypotensive effects, especially in the presence of one or more predisposing factors such as significant renal impairment, severe diabetes, potassium supplements, high potassium diet, and advanced age. Other drugs that may exhibit hyperkalemic activity include **ARBs inhibitors, drospirenone** (Yasmin), **heparins, nonselective beta-blockers, NSAIDs, COX-2 inhibitors, cyclosporine, tacrolimus, succinylcholine, pentamidine, trimethoprim,** and **potassium-containing salt substitutes**. The product information states that aliskiren is contraindicated in patients with diabetes who are receiving ACE inhibitors.

CLASS 3: ASSESS RISK & TAKE ACTION IF NECESSARY
* *Monitor*: Monitor serum potassium concentrations and blood pressure, especially in patients with predisposing factors such as renal disease, diabetes, and advanced age.

OBJECT DRUGS		PRECIPITANT DRUGS
Angiotensin Receptor Blockers (ARBs):		**Tizanidine** (Zanaflex)
Azilsartan (Edarbi)	**Losartan** (Cozaar)	
Candesartan (Atacand)	**Olmesartan** (Benicar)	
Eprosartan (Teveten)	**Telmisartan** (Micardis)	
Irbesartan (Avapro)	**Valsartan** (Diovan)	

COMMENTS: Patients on ACE inhibitors have developed severe hypotension after starting tizanidine therapy; theoretically, a similar reaction could occur if tizanidine were added to ARB therapy. Tizanidine, like the antihypertensive drug clonidine, is an alpha-2 adrenergic agonist, and may have additive hypotensive effects with ARBs.

CLASS 3: ASSESS RISK & TAKE ACTION IF NECESSARY
* *Consider Alternative*: In patients taking an ARB, consider using muscle relaxants other than tizanidine (that are not alpha-2 adrenergic agonists). Some other muscle relaxants can also sometimes cause hypotension, but the risk is probably less than for tizanidine.
* *Monitor*: If tizanidine is used in a patient taking an ARB, monitor cardiovascular status carefully for evidence of an acute hypotensive reaction.

OBJECT DRUGS	PRECIPITANT DRUGS	
Antiarrhythmics (CYP3A4 Substrates):	**Antimicrobials:**	
Amiodarone (Cordarone)	**Ciprofloxacin** (Cipro)	**Posaconazole** (Noxafil)
Disopyramide (Norpace)	**Clarithromycin** (Biaxin)	**Quinupristin** (Synercid)
Dronedarone (Multaq)	**Erythromycin** (E-Mycin)	**Telithromycin** (Ketek)
Quinidine (Quinidex)	**Fluconazole** (Diflucan)	**Troleandomycin** (TAO)
	Itraconazole (Sporanox)	**Voriconazole** (Vfend)
	Ketoconazole (Nizoral)	

COMMENTS: Although data are limited, any CYP3A4 inhibitor could increase the plasma concentrations of these antiarrhythmic drugs. Toxicity including cardiac arrhythmias could result. Assume that all CYP3A4 inhibitors interact until proven otherwise.

CLASS 3: ASSESS RISK & TAKE ACTION IF NECESSARY
- *Consider Alternative*:
  Azole Antifungals: Fluconazole appears to be a less potent inhibitor of CYP3A4 than itraconazole or ketoconazole, but in larger doses it also inhibits CYP3A4. **Terbinafine** (Lamisil) does not appear to affect CYP3A4.
  Macrolide Antibiotics: Unlike erythromycin, clarithromycin and troleandomycin, other macrolides such as **azithromycin** (Zithromax) and **dirithromycin*** do not appear to inhibit CYP3A4. (*not available in US)
  Telithromycin: The use of **azithromycin** (Zithromax) or a quinolone antibiotic other than ciprofloxacin should be considered.
- *Monitor*: Monitor for altered antiarrhythmic response if the CYP3A4 inhibitor is initiated, discontinued, or changed in dosage. Monitor for ECG changes indicating antiarrhythmic toxicity, and measure antiarrhythmic plasma concentrations as needed.

OBJECT DRUGS	PRECIPITANT DRUGS
Antiarrhythmics	**Antidepressants:**
(CYP3A4 Substrates):	**Fluvoxamine** (Luvox)
Amiodarone (Cordarone)	**Nefazodone**
Disopyramide (Norpace)	
Dronedarone (Multaq)	
Quinidine (Quinidex)	

COMMENTS: Although data are limited, antidepressants that inhibit CYP3A4 could increase the plasma concentrations of these antiarrhythmics. Toxicity including cardiac arrhythmias could result. Assume that all CYP3A4 inhibitors interact until proven otherwise.

CLASS 3: ASSESS RISK & TAKE ACTION IF NECESSARY
- *Consider Alternative*:
  Antidepressants: Citalopram (Celexa), **desvenlafaxine** (Pristiq), **escitalopram** (Lexapro), **paroxetine** (Paxil), **sertraline** (Zoloft), and **venlafaxine** (Effexor) appear to have minimal effects on CYP3A4. **Fluoxetine** (Prozac) appears to be a weak inhibitor of CYP3A4.
- *Monitor*: Monitor for altered antiarrhythmic response if the CYP3A4 inhibitor is initiated, discontinued, or changed in dosage. Monitor for ECG changes indicating antiarrhythmic toxicity, and measure antiarrhythmic plasma concentrations as needed.

OBJECT DRUGS	PRECIPITANT DRUGS
Antiarrhythmics (CYP3A4 Substrates):	**Calcium Channel Blockers:**
Amiodarone (Cordarone)	**Diltiazem** (Cardizem)
Disopyramide (Norpace)	**Verapamil** (Isoptin)
Dronedarone (Multaq)	
Quinidine (Quinidex)	

COMMENTS: Although data are limited, any calcium channel blocker that inhibits CYP3A4 could increase the plasma concentrations of these antiarrhythmic drugs. Toxicity including cardiac arrhythmias could result. Assume that all CYP3A4 inhibitors interact until proven otherwise.

CLASS 3: ASSESS RISK & TAKE ACTION IF NECESSARY
- *Consider Alternative*:
  Calcium Channel Blockers: Calcium channel blockers other than diltiazem and verapamil are unlikely to inhibit the metabolism of these antiarrhythmics.
- *Monitor*: Monitor for altered antiarrhythmic response if the CYP3A4 inhibitor is initiated, discontinued, or changed in dosage. Monitor for ECG changes indicating antiarrhythmic toxicity, and measure antiarrhythmic plasma concentrations as needed.

OBJECT DRUGS	PRECIPITANT DRUGS	
Antiarrhythmics	**Enzyme Inhibitors:**	
(CYP3A4 Substrates):	**Amiodarone** (Cordarone)	**Delavirdine** (Rescriptor)
Amiodarone (Cordarone)	**Amprenavir** (Agenerase)	**Dronedarone** (Multaq)
Disopyramide (Norpace)	**Aprepitant** (Emend)	**Grapefruit**
Dronedarone (Multaq)	**Atazanavir** (Reyataz)	**Indinavir** (Crixivan)
Quinidine (Quinidex)	**Boceprevir** (Victrelis)	**Lomitapide** (Juxtapid)
	Ceritinib (Zykadia)	**Mifepristone** (Korlym)
	Cobicistat (Stribild)	**Nelfinavir** (Viracept)
	Conivaptan (Vaprisol)	**Ritonavir** (Norvir)
	Cyclosporine (Neoral)	**Saquinavir** (Invirase)
	Darunavir (Prezista)	**Telaprevir** (Incivek)

COMMENTS: Although data are limited, any CYP3A4 inhibitor could increase the plasma concentrations of these antiarrhythmic drugs. Toxicity including cardiac arrhythmias could result. Assume that all CYP3A4 inhibitors interact until proven otherwise. The mifepristone product information states that concurrent use of quinidine is contraindicated.

CLASS 3: ASSESS RISK & TAKE ACTION IF NECESSARY
- *Consider Alternative*:
  Grapefruit: Orange juice does not appear to inhibit CYP3A4.
- *Monitor*: Monitor for altered antiarrhythmic response if the CYP3A4 inhibitor is initiated, discontinued, or changed in dosage. Monitor for ECG changes indicating antiarrhythmic toxicity, and measure antiarrhythmic plasma concentrations as needed.

OBJECT DRUGS	PRECIPITANT DRUGS	
Antiarrhythmics	**Enzyme Inducers:**	
(CYP3A4 Substrates):	**Barbiturates**	**Oxcarbazepine** (Trileptal)
Amiodarone (Cordarone)	**Bosentan** (Tracleer)	**Phenytoin** (Dilantin)
Disopyramide (Norpace)	**Carbamazepine** (Tegretol)	**Primidone** (Mysoline)
Dronedarone (Multaq)	**Dabrafenib** (Tafinlar)	**Rifabutin** (Mycobutin)
Quinidine (Quinidex)	**Dexamethasone** (Decadron)	**Rifampin** (Rifadin)
	Efavirenz (Sustiva)	**Rifapentine** (Priftin)
	Lumacaftor (Orkambi)	**St. John's wort**
	Nevirapine (Viramune)	

COMMENTS: CYP3A4 is quite sensitive to enzyme induction, and enzyme inducers have been shown to reduce plasma concentrations of these antiarrhythmic drugs. Depending on the potency of the enzyme inducer, the reductions in antiarrhythmic plasma concentrations may result in substantial reductions in antiarrhythmic effects. Note also that some of these antiarrhythmics inhibit various enzyme and transporters (see CYP table), and may affect the plasma concentrations of the enzyme inducer. It has also been proposed that amiodarone is converted to hepatotoxic metabolites by CYP3A4; thus, inducers of CYP3A4 might increase the hepatotoxicity of amiodarone.

CLASS 3: ASSESS RISK & TAKE ACTION IF NECESSARY
- *Consider Alternative*:
  St. John's wort: Given the limited evidence of efficacy, St. John's wort should generally be avoided in patients taking one of these antiarrhythmic agents.
- *Monitor*: Monitor for altered antiarrhythmic response if the CYP3A4 inducer is initiated, discontinued, or changed in dosage. Monitor for ECG changes indicating loss of antiarrhythmic efficacy, and measure antiarrhythmic plasma concentrations as needed. Note that the effect of enzyme inducers is often gradual, and it can take up to 1 to 2 weeks for maximal effects, and from 1 to 4 weeks for the effect to dissipate (depending on which inducer is used).

OBJECT DRUGS	PRECIPITANT DRUGS
Antiarrhythmics	**Antidepressants:**
(CYP2D6 Substrates:	**Bupropion** (Wellbutrin)
Flecainide (Tambocor)	**Duloxetine** (Cymbalta)
Mexiletine (Mexitil)	**Fluoxetine** (Prozac)
Propafenone (Rythmol)	**Paroxetine** (Paxil)

COMMENTS: These antidepressants inhibit CYP2D6, and can lead to accumulation of flecainide, mexiletine, or propafenone, and may increase the risk of toxicity. People with "normal" CYP2D6 activity (Extensive Metabolizers) are at the greatest risk.

CLASS 2: USE ONLY IF BENEFIT FELT TO OUTWEIGH RISK
- *Use Alternative*:
  Antidepressant: **Citalopram** (Celexa), **desvenlafaxine** (Pristiq), **escitalopram** (Lexapro), and **sertraline** (Zoloft), are weak inhibitors of CYP2D6, and **fluvoxamine** and **venlafaxine** (Effexor) have little or no effect on CYP2D6.
- *Monitor*: Be alert for an increased effect of the antiarrhythmic if CYP2D6 inhibitors are coadministered. Monitoring of the antiarrhythmic plasma concentration is warranted.

OBJECT DRUGS	PRECIPITANT DRUGS	
Antiarrhythmics	**Enzyme Inhibitors:**	
(CYP2D6 Substrates:	**Abiraterone** (Zytiga)	**Propoxyphene***
Flecainide (Tambocor)	**Amiodarone** (Cordarone)	**Quinidine** (Quinidex)
Mexiletine (Mexitil)	**Cinacalcet** (Sensipar)	**Ritonavir** (Norvir)
Propafenone (Rythmol)	**Clobazam** (Onfi)	**Terbinafine** (Lamisil)
	Diphenhydramine (Benadryl)	**Thioridazine** (Mellaril)
	Haloperidol (Haldol)	
	Mirabegron (Myrbetriq)	
	Propafenone (Rythmol)	

* Propoxyphene (Darvon) was withdrawn from the US market.

COMMENTS: Drugs that inhibit CYP2D6 can lead to accumulation of flecainide, mexiletine, and propafenone, and increase the risk of toxicity. People with "normal" CYP2D6 activity (Extensive Metabolizers) are at the greatest risk. Note that because terbinafine has an extraordinarily long terminal half-life, the inhibitory effect of terbinafine on CYP2D6 may last for many weeks after terbinafine is discontinued.

CLASS 2: USE ONLY IF BENEFIT FELT TO OUTWEIGH RISK
- *Use Alternative*:
  Diphenhydramine: Other antihistamines such as **desloratadine** (Clarinex), **fexofenadine** (Allegra), **loratadine** Claritin), and **cetirizine** (Zyrtec) are not known to inhibit CYP2D6.
- *Monitor*: Be alert for an increased effect of the antiarrhythmic if CYP2D6 inhibitors are coadministered. Monitoring of the antiarrhythmic plasma concentration is warranted.

OBJECT DRUGS	PRECIPITANT DRUGS
Anticoagulants, Oral:	**Analgesics:**
Acenocoumarol	**Acetaminophen** (Tylenol)
Phenprocoumon	**Aspirin**
Warfarin (Coumadin)	

COMMENTS: Aspirin increases the risk of bleeding in anticoagulated patients due to inhibition of platelet function and gastric erosions. Large doses of aspirin (e.g. 3g/day or more) can increase the hypoprothrombinemic response. However, low (antiplatelet) doses of aspirin appear to increase primarily minor bleeding and the combination is used intentionally in many patients. In some patients, acetaminophen can increase the hypoprothrombinemic response to warfarin and probably other oral anticoagulants. In most cases the interaction is small, but in predisposed patients marked hypoprothrombinemia has been reported. It would be prudent to limit acetaminophen dosage to 2 g/day or less for no more than a few days, and to monitor the INR.

CLASS 2: USE ONLY IF BENEFIT FELT TO OUTWEIGH RISK
- *Use Alternative*: As an analgesic, acetaminophen appears safer than aspirin for patients on warfarin (but avoid large or prolonged doses of acetaminophen). If a NSAID is required, see Anticoagulants, Oral + NSAIDs. Most opiates appear to have little effect on the anticoagulant response to warfarin, but there are case reports of increased warfarin effect due to **tramadol** (Ultram).
- *Circumvent/Minimize*: Advise patients on oral anticoagulants to avoid taking acetaminophen, aspirin or other salicylates unless instructed to do so by the prescriber of the oral anticoagulant.

- **Monitor:** Monitor the INR if acetaminophen or large doses of salicylates are given for more than a few days. Note that the increased bleeding risk from small doses of aspirin (e.g., less than 2 to 3 g/day) is usually not reflected in an increased INR or prothrombin time. Monitor carefully for clinical evidence of bleeding, especially from the gastrointestinal tract.

OBJECT DRUGS	PRECIPITANT DRUGS
Anticoagulants, Oral:	**Absorption Inhibitors:**
Acenocoumarol	**Cholestyramine** (Questran)
Phenprocoumon	**Colestipol** (Colestid)
Warfarin (Coumadin)	**Sucralfate** (Carafate)

COMMENTS: Bile acid binding resins and sucralfate bind with warfarin, phenprocoumon, and possibly other oral anticoagulants in the G.I. tract, thus reducing the anticoagulant absorption and response. Since warfarin and phenprocoumon undergo enterohepatic circulation, the binding cannot be completely avoided by spacing doses of the drugs.

CLASS 3: ASSESS RISK & TAKE ACTION IF NECESSARY
- **Circumvent/Minimize:** Give oral anticoagulants 2 hours before or 6 hours after absorption inhibitors; keep constant interval between doses of oral anticoagulant and absorption inhibitor.
- **Consider Alternative: Ezetimibe** (Zetia) does not appear to affect the bioavailability of warfarin. The manufacturer found that **colesevelam** (WelChol) did not affect warfarin plasma concentrations, but they have received isolated reports of decreased INR when colesevelam was used with warfarin. More study is needed.
- **Monitor:** Monitor response to anticoagulant if absorption inhibitor is initiated, discontinued, changed in dosage or if the interval between doses of the oral anticoagulant and the absorption inhibitor is changed.

OBJECT DRUGS	PRECIPITANT DRUGS	
Anticoagulants, Oral:	**Enzyme Inducers:**	
Acenocoumarol	**Azathioprine** (Imuran)	**Oxcarbazepine** (Trileptal)
Phenprocoumon	**Barbiturates**	**Phenytoin** (Dilantin)
Warfarin (Coumadin)	**Bosentan** (Tracleer)	**Primidone** (Mysoline)
	Carbamazepine (Tegretol)	**Rifabutin** (Mycobutin)
	Cloxacillin (Cloxapen)	**Rifampin** (Rifadin)
	Dabrafenib (Tafinlar)	**Rifapentine** (Priftin)
	Dicloxacillin (Dynapen)	**St. John's wort**
	Griseofulvin (Grisactin)	
	Nafcillin (Unipen)	

COMMENTS: Enzyme inducers gradually reduce the anticoagulant response to oral anticoagulants. Phenytoin may actually *increase* warfarin effect initially—possibly by competitively inhibiting CYP2C9 activity and displacement of warfarin from plasma protein binding—but the initial increase is followed by reduced anticoagulant effect due to enzyme induction. Consider the increased risk of impaired anticoagulant control, and the increased monitoring cost, especially if the enzyme inducer will *not* be used chronically in a stable dose. Azathioprine appears to inhibit the anticoagulant effect of warfarin, but the mechanism for this effect is not clear. Theoretically, mercaptopurine may produce a similar effect on warfarin.

CLASS 2: USE ONLY IF BENEFIT FELT TO OUTWEIGH RISK
- **Use Alternative:**
  General: Suitable alternatives with equivalent efficacy are not available for most enzyme inducers. In patients stabilized on chronic therapy with the anticoagulant and an enzyme inducer, it may be better to maintain current therapy, making sure the patient knows not to stop or change the dose of the enzyme inducer without consulting the prescriber of the anticoagulant.
  St. John's wort: Given the limited evidence of efficacy, St. John's wort should generally be avoided in patients taking oral anticoagulants.
- **Monitor:** If it is necessary to use enzyme inducers and oral anticoagulants concurrently, monitor for altered response if the inducer is initiated, discontinued, or changed in dosage. Note that enzyme induction is often gradual; it can take up to 1 to 2 weeks or more for maximal effects, and from 1 to 4 weeks for the effect to dissipate (depending on which inducer is used).

7

OBJECT DRUGS	PRECIPITANT DRUGS
Anticoagulants, Oral:	**Enzyme Inhibitors:**
Acenocoumarol	Alcohol (intoxication)
Warfarin (Coumadin)	Sulfinpyrazone (Anturane)

COMMENTS: Acute alcohol intoxication can markedly increase the effect of warfarin. Azapropazone and sulfinpyrazone markedly increase the anticoagulant response to warfarin, due primarily to inhibition of CYP2C9 (assume that acenocoumarol interacts similarly until proved otherwise).

CLASS 1: AVOID COMBINATION
- *Avoid*: Patients receiving oral anticoagulants should avoid alcohol intoxication, but available evidence suggests that modest alcohol intake (e.g., 1-2 drinks/day) has little or no effect on warfarin response. Since azapropazone and sulfinpyrazone can markedly increase warfarin response, concurrent use should be avoided.

OBJECT DRUGS	PRECIPITANT DRUGS
Anticoagulants, Oral:	**HMG CoA Reductase Inhibitors:**
Acenocoumarol	Fluvastatin (Lescol)
Warfarin (Coumadin)	Lovastatin (Mevacor)
	Rosuvastatin (Crestor)
	Simvastatin (Zocor)

COMMENTS: Fluvastatin, and to a lesser degree, lovastatin and simvastatin, inhibit CYP2C9 and may increase the hypoprothrombinemic response to warfarin in some patients. Rosuvastatin has been noted to increase the INR in patients taking warfarin.

CLASS 3: ASSESS RISK & TAKE ACTION IF NECESSARY
- *Consider Alternative*: Other HMG CoA reductase inhibitors such as **pitavastatin** (Livalo), **pravastatin** (Pravachol) and **atorvastatin** (Lipitor) appear to have little or no effect on warfarin response.
- *Monitor*: Monitor for altered warfarin response if fluvastatin, lovastatin, rosuvastatin, or simvastatin are initiated, discontinued, or changed in dosage.

OBJECT DRUGS	PRECIPITANT DRUGS
Anticoagulants, Oral:	**Azole Antifungals:**
Acenocoumarol	Fluconazole (Diflucan)
Warfarin (Coumadin)	Miconazole (Monistat)
	Voriconazole (Vfend)

COMMENTS: Fluconazole is a potent inhibitor of CYP2C9, and even at a dose of 100 mg/day can substantially increase the hypoprothrombinemic response of warfarin. Miconazole also strongly inhibits S-warfarin metabolism. Several cases have been reported of marked increase in warfarin effect following the use of miconazole oral gel, probably because the oral gel was swallowed and absorbed. Vaginal miconazole has also increased warfarin response in isolated cases. Topical administration of miconazole on the skin has been reported to increase warfarin effect, but the effect appears to be rare.

CLASS 2: USE ONLY IF BENEFIT FELT TO OUTWEIGH RISK
- *Use Alternative*: Itraconazole (Sporanox), **ketoconazole** (Nizoral), **posaconazole** (Noxafil), and **terbinafine** (Lamisil) probably have less effect on warfarin metabolism than other azole antifungals. Nonetheless, isolated cases of increased warfarin effect have been reported, and one should still monitor for increased warfarin response.
- *Monitor*: Monitor for altered hypoprothrombinemic response if an azole antifungal is initiated, discontinued, or changed in dosage.

OBJECT DRUGS	PRECIPITANT DRUGS
Anticoagulants, Oral: **Acenocoumarol** **Warfarin** (Coumadin)	**Cimetidine** (Tagamet)

COMMENTS: Cimetidine increases the hypoprothrombinemic response to warfarin. Although the effect is usually modest, it is also highly variable from patient to patient; hence, an occasional patient may develop a substantial increase in warfarin response.

CLASS 3: ASSESS RISK & TAKE ACTION IF NECESSARY
- *Consider Alternative*: Other acid suppressors are unlikely to interact. Consider using **famotidine** (Pepcid), **nizatidine** (Axid), **ranitidine** (Zantac), **dexlansoprazole** (Kapidex), **lansoprazole** (Prevacid), **rabeprazole** (Aciphex), **omeprazole** (Prilosec), **esomeprazole** (Nexium), or **pantoprazole** (Protonix).
- *Monitor*: If the combination is used, monitor for altered warfarin response when cimetidine is initiated, discontinued, or changed in dosage.

OBJECT DRUGS	PRECIPITANT DRUGS
Anticoagulants, Oral: **Acenocoumarol** **Warfarin** (Coumadin)	**Antibiotics:** **Chloramphenicol** (Chloromycetin) **Co-trimoxazole** (Septra) **Metronidazole** (Flagyl) **Sulfamethizole** (Urobiotic) **Sulfaphenazole**

COMMENTS: Sulfamethoxazole (eg, co-trimoxazole) and metronidazole are known inhibitors of CYP2C9 and can substantially increase warfarin plasma concentrations and hypoprothrombinemic response. The ability of chloramphenicol to inhibit CYP2C9 is based primarily on theoretical considerations. Many other antibiotics have been reported to increase warfarin response in isolated case reports, but these reports can be difficult to evaluate because such patients may have other risk factors for increased warfarin effect such as fever, poor oral intake, and acute illness. (See the Table **Effect of Other Antibiotics on Warfarin** at the end of the monographs.) Epidemiologic studies suggest that patients on warfarin who receive *any* antibiotic may be at increased risk for gastrointestinal bleeding.

CLASS 2: USE ONLY IF BENEFIT FELT TO OUTWEIGH RISK
- *Use Alternative*: Almost all antibiotics have been associated with increased warfarin response in at least a few patients, but most of them appear less likely to interact with warfarin than the antibiotics listed above.
- *Monitor*: If one of the antibiotics listed above must be used in a patient on warfarin, monitor anticoagulation carefully; an adjustment in warfarin dosage may be needed. Other antibiotics appear less likely to interact, but one should still monitor for altered effect.

OBJECT DRUGS	PRECIPITANT DRUGS
Anticoagulants, Oral: **Acenocoumarol** **Warfarin** (Coumadin)	**Antidepressants:** **Fluoxetine** (Prozac) **Fluvoxamine** (Luvox)

COMMENTS: CYP2C9 inhibitors increase S-warfarin concentrations; the onset of increased anticoagulant effect is usually gradual (over 7-10 days). Most studies involve warfarin, but assume that acenocoumarol interacts similarly until proved otherwise. Phenprocoumon is metabolized primarily by glucuronidation and theoretically would be unlikely to interact with CYP2C9 inhibitors. Also, SSRIs as a class may increase the risk of bleeding in patients receiving oral anticoagulants, even in the absence of a pharmacokinetic interaction.

CLASS 2: USE ONLY IF BENEFIT FELT TO OUTWEIGH RISK
- *Use Alternative*: Other SSRIs such as **citalopram** (Celexa), **escitalopram** (Lexapro), **desvenlafaxine** (Pristiq), **venlafaxine** (Effexor), **paroxetine** (Paxil) or **sertraline** (Zoloft) may be less likely to increase the hypoprothrombinemic response to warfarin, but SSRIs may increase bleeding risk even in the absence of increased INR response due to their antiplatelet effects.
- *Monitor*: Monitor for altered anticoagulant effect if fluvoxamine or fluoxetine is initiated, discontinued, or changed in dosage.

9

OBJECT DRUGS	PRECIPITANT DRUGS	
Anticoagulants, Oral:	**Enzyme Inhibitors:**	
Acenocoumarol	**Amiodarone** (Cordarone)	**Gemfibrozil** (Lopid)
Warfarin (Coumadin)	**Androgens**	**Imatinib** (Gleevec)
	Capecitabine (Xeloda)	**Leflunomide** (Arava)
	Ceritinib (Zykadia)	**Lomitapide** (Juxtapid)
	Danazol (Danocrine)	**Mefloquine** (Lariam)
	Disulfiram (Antabuse)	**Tamoxifen** (Nolvadex)
	Etravirine (Intelence)	**Valproic Acid** (Depakote)
	Fenofibrate (Tricor)	**Zafirlukast** (Accolate)
	Fluorouracil (5-FU)	

COMMENTS: CYP2C9 inhibitors increase S-warfarin concentrations; the increased anticoagulant effect is usually gradual (over 7-10 days). The interaction magnitude varies considerably from patient to patient, and is usually dose related. Amiodarone may also increase oral anticoagulant response by increasing circulating thyroid hormone concentrations. The mechanism for the effect of androgens, danazol, and fibrates (clofibrate, fenofibrate, gemfibrozil) on warfarin response is not established. The leflunomide-warfarin interaction is based on limited clinical information. Most studies involve warfarin, but assume that acenocoumarol interacts similarly until proved otherwise. **Phenprocoumon** is primarily glucuronidated; it is unlikely to interact with CYP2C9 inhibitors.

CLASS 2: USE ONLY IF BENEFIT FELT TO OUTWEIGH RISK
- *Use Alternative*:
  Zafirlukast: **Montelukast** (Singulair) does not appear to interact with warfarin. **Zileuton** (Zyflo) may increase warfarin response somewhat, but probably to a lesser extent than zafirlukast.
- *Monitor*: If a CYP2C9 inhibitor is used, monitor for altered anticoagulant effect if inhibitor is initiated, discontinued, or changed in dosage. Amiodarone-induced inhibition may require several weeks to develop.

OBJECT DRUGS	PRECIPITANT DRUGS	
Anticoagulants, Oral:	**NSAIDs:**	
Acenocoumarol	**Diclofenac** (Voltaren)	**Meclofenamate**
Phenprocoumon	**Diflunisal** (Dolobid)	**Mefenamic acid**
Warfarin (Coumadin)	**Etodolac** (Lodine)	**Meloxicam** (Mobic)
	Fenoprofen (Nalfon)	**Nabumetone** (Relafen)
	Flurbiprofen (Ansaid)	**Naproxen** (Aleve)
	Ibuprofen (Motrin)	**Oxaprozin** (Daypro)
	Indomethacin (Indocin)	**Piroxicam** (Feldene)
	Ketoprofen (Orudis)	**Sulindac** (Clinoril)
	Ketorolac (Toradol)	**Tolmetin** (Tolectin)

COMMENTS: All NSAIDs reversibly inhibit platelet function and cause gastric erosions. The risk of GI bleeding appears to be considerably increased with NSAIDs plus warfarin compared to either drug used alone. Some NSAIDs can increase the hypoprothrombinemic response to oral anticoagulants.

CLASS 2: USE ONLY IF BENEFIT FELT TO OUTWEIGH RISK
- *Use Alternative*: Use a non-NSAID analgesic if possible such as acetaminophen (see Acetaminophen discussion under Anticoagulants, Oral + Aspirin). If a NSAID is required, non-acetylated salicylates such as **choline magnesium trisalicylate** (Trilisate), **magnesium salicylates**, and **salsalate** (Disalcid) are probably safer due to minimal effects on platelets and gastric mucosa; if large doses are used, monitor INR. COX-2 inhibitors produce no platelet inhibition and probably less gastric damage. Studies indicate that celecoxib does not affect warfarin response. However, isolated case reports of warfarin interactions with celecoxib have appeared, and epidemiologic evidence suggests that COX-2 inhibitors may increase the risk of upper GI hemorrhage in patients on warfarin. If a standard NSAID is used, consider using NSAIDs that are unlikely to affect the hypoprothrombinemic response such as diclofenac, ibuprofen, naproxen, and tolmetin.
- *Monitor*: If any NSAID is used with an oral anticoagulant, monitor carefully for evidence of bleeding, especially from the GI tract.

10

OBJECT DRUGS	PRECIPITANT DRUGS	
Anticoagulants, Oral:	**Antimicrobials:**	
Apixaban (Eliquis)	**Ciprofloxacin** (Cipro)	**Ketoconazole** (Nizoral)
Rivaroxaban (Xarelto)	**Clarithromycin** (Biaxin)	**Posaconazole** (Noxafil)
	Erythromycin (E-Mycin)	**Quinupristin** (Synercid)
	Fluconazole (Diflucan)	**Telithromycin** (Ketek)
	Isoniazid (INH)	**Troleandomycin** (TAO)
	Itraconazole (Sporanox)	**Voriconazole** (Vfend)

COMMENTS: These antimicrobials inhibit CYP3A4 and may increase the plasma concentration of apixaban and rivaroxaban. Since apixaban and rivaroxaban are also substrates for P-glycoprotein, precipitant drugs that inhibit both CYP3A4 and P-glycoprotein may produce a larger increase in anticoagulant concentrations.

CLASS 3: ASSESS RISK & TAKE ACTION IF NECESSARY
* *Consider Alternative*:
  Azole Antifungals: Fluconazole appears to be a less potent inhibitor of CYP3A4; but in larger doses it also inhibits CYP3A4. **Terbinafine** (Lamisil) does not appear to affect CYP3A4. Macrolide Antibiotics: **Azithromycin** (Zithromax) and **dirithromycin*** do not appear to inhibit CYP3A4 and are unlikely to interact. (*not available in US).
* *Monitor*: Monitor for altered rivaroxaban effect if one of these antimicrobials is initiated, discontinued or changed in dosage; adjustments of rivaroxaban dosage may be needed. If rivaroxaban is initiated in the presence of therapy with one of these agents, consider conservative doses of rivaroxaban.

OBJECT DRUGS	PRECIPITANT DRUGS	
Anticoagulants, Oral:	**Enzyme Inducers:**	
Apixaban (Eliquis)	**Barbiturates**	**Oxcarbazepine** (Trileptal)
Rivaroxaban (Xarelto)	**Bosentan** (Tracleer)	**Phenytoin** (Dilantin)
	Carbamazepine (Tegretol)	**Primidone** (Mysoline)
	Dabrafenib (Tafinlar)	**Rifabutin** (Mycobutin)
	Efavirenz (Sustiva)	**Rifampin** (Rifadin)
	Lumacaftor (Orkambi)	**Rifapentine** (Priftin)
	Etravirine (Intelence)	**St. John's wort**
	Nevirapine (Viramune)	

COMMENTS: Inducers of CYP3A4 may reduce the concentration of apixaban and rivaroxaban. Several days to weeks may be required to see the full effect an inducer on apixaban or rivaroxaban. Since apixaban and rivaroxaban are also substrates for P-glycoprotein, precipitant drugs that induce both CYP3A4 and P-glycoprotein may produce a larger decrease in anticoagulant concentrations. A reduction in the anticoagulant effect may occur.

CLASS 3: ASSESS RISK & TAKE ACTION IF NECESSARY
Monitor: Monitor for altered anticoagulant effect if a CYP3A4 or P-glycoprotein inducer is initiated, discontinued or changed in dosage; adjustments of anticoagulant dosage may be needed.

11

OBJECT DRUGS	PRECIPITANT DRUGS
Anticoagulants, Oral:	**P-glycoprotein Inducers:**
Apixaban (Eliquis)	**Carbamazepine** (Tegretol)
Dabigatran (Pradaxa)	**Dexamethasone** (Decadron)
Rivaroxaban (Xarelto)	**Rifampin** (Rimactane)
	St. John's wort
	Tipranavir (Aptivus)

COMMENTS: Rifampin has been reported to markedly reduce the plasma concentration of dabigatran. Other P-glycoprotein inducers are likely to have a similar effect on these anticoagulants. Several days to weeks may be required to see the full effect a P-glycoprotein inducer on the anticoagulant. Since apixaban and rivaroxaban are also substrates for CYP3A4, precipitant drugs that induce both CYP3A4 and P-glycoprotein may produce a larger decrease in anticoagulant concentrations.

CLASS 3: ASSESS RISK & TAKE ACTION IF NECESSARY
Monitor: Monitor for altered anticoagulant effect if a P-glycoprotein inducer is initiated, discontinued or changed in dosage; adjustments of anticoagulant dosage may be needed.

OBJECT DRUGS	PRECIPITANT DRUGS	
Anticoagulants, Oral:	**P-glycoprotein Inhibitors:**	
Apixaban (Eliquis)	**Amiodarone** (Cordarone)	**Nelfinavir** (Viracept)
Dabigatran (Pradaxa)	**Azithromycin** (Zithromax)	**Paritaprevir** (Technivie)
Rivaroxaban (Xarelto)	**Clarithromycin** (Biaxin)	**Posaconazole** (Noxafil)
	Conivaptan (Vaprisol)	**Propafenone** (Rythmol)
	Cyclosporine (Neoral)	**Quinidine** (Quinidex)
	Daclatasvir (Daklinza)	**Ranolazine** (Ranexa)
	Dronedarone (Multaq)	**Ritonavir** (Norvir)
	Erythromycin (E-Mycin)	**Saquinavir** (Invirase)
	Hydroxychloroquine	**Sunitinib** (Sutent)
	Indinavir (Crixivan)	**Tacrolimus** (Prograf)
	Itraconazole (Sporanox)	**Tamoxifen** (Nolvadex)
	Ketoconazole (Nizoral)	**Telaprevir** (Incivek)
	Ledipasvir (Harvoni)	**Telithromycin** (Ketek)

COMMENTS: Inhibitors of P-glycoprotein increase the absorption of the pro-drug dabigatran etexilate, potentially increasing the concentration of the active drug dabigatran. Since P-glycoprotein inhibitors can increase the concentration of these anticoagulants; monitor for increased anticoagulation effects.

CLASS 3: ASSESS RISK & TAKE ACTION IF NECESSARY
- *Circumvent/Minimize*: Administration of dabigatran at least 2 hours before the P-glycoprotein inhibitor should minimize the effect on the absorption of dabigatran etexilate.
- *Monitor*: Monitor for altered anticoagulant effect if one of these P-glycoprotein inhibitors is initiated, discontinued or changed in dosage; adjustments of anticoagulant dosage may be needed.

12

OBJECT DRUGS	PRECIPITANT DRUGS	
Anticoagulants, Oral:	**Enzyme Inhibitors:**	
Apixaban (Eliquis)	**Amiodarone** (Cordarone)	**Delavirdine** (Rescriptor)
Rivaroxaban (Xarelto)	**Amprenavir** (Agenerase)	**Dronedarone** (Multaq)
	Aprepitant (Emend)	**Indinavir** (Crixivan)
	Atazanavir (Reyataz)	**Lomitapide** (Juxtapid)
	Boceprevir (Victrelis)	**Mifepristone** (Korlym)
	Ceritinib (Zykadia)	**Nefazodone**
	Cobicistat (Stribild)	**Nelfinavir** (Viracept)
	Conivaptan (Vaprisol)	**Ritonavir** (Norvir)
	Cyclosporine (Neoral)	**Saquinavir** (Invirase)
	Danazol (Danocrine)	**Tamoxifen** (Nolvadex)
	Darunavir (Prezista)	**Telaprevir** (Incivek)

COMMENTS: These precipitant drugs inhibit CYP3A4 and may increase the plasma concentration of apixaban and rivaroxaban. Since apixaban and rivaroxaban are also substrates for P-glycoprotein, precipitant drugs that inhibit both CYP3A4 and P-glycoprotein may produce a larger increase in anticoagulant concentrations.

CLASS 3: ASSESS RISK & TAKE ACTION IF NECESSARY
• *Monitor:* Monitor for altered anticoagulant effect if one of these inhibitors is initiated, discontinued or changed in dosage; adjustments of anticoagulant dosage may be needed. If the anticoagulant is initiated in the presence of therapy with one of these agents, consider initiating therapy with conservative doses of anticoagulant.

OBJECT DRUGS	PRECIPITANT DRUGS
Anticoagulants, Oral:	**Calcium Channel Blockers:**
Apixaban (Eliquis)	**Bepridil** (Vascor)
Dabigatran (Pradaxa)	**Diltiazem** (Cardizem)
Rivaroxaban (Xarelto)	**Verapamil** (Isoptin)

COMMENTS: Inhibitors of P-glycoprotein may increase the concentration of the anticoagulant. Since apixaban and rivaroxaban are also substrates for CYP3A4, precipitant drugs that inhibit both CYP3A4 and P-glycoprotein may produce a larger increase in anticoagulant concentrations.

CLASS 3: ASSESS RISK & TAKE ACTION IF NECESSARY
• *Consider Alternative:* Dihydropyridine calcium channel blockers such as **felodipine** (Plendil) or **nifedipine** (Procardia) do not appear to inhibit CYP3A4 or P-glycoprotein and would not be expected to alter anticoagulant concentrations.
• *Monitor:* Monitor for altered anticoagulant effect if one of these calcium channel blockers is initiated, discontinued or changed in dosage; adjustments of anticoagulant dosage may be needed. If the anticoagulant is initiated in the presence of therapy with one of these agents, consider conservative doses of anticoagulant.

OBJECT DRUGS	PRECIPITANT DRUGS	
Antidepressants, Tricyclic:	**Enzyme Inducers:**	
Amitriptyline (Elavil)	**Barbiturates**	**Phenytoin** (Dilantin)
Amoxapine (Asendin)	**Bosentan** (Tracleer)	**Primidone** (Mysoline)
Clomipramine (Anafranil)	**Carbamazepine** (Tegretol)	**Rifabutin** (Mycobutin)
Desipramine (Norpramin)	**Dabrafenib** (Tafinlar)	**Rifampin** (Rifadin)
Doxepin (Sinequan)	**Dexamethasone** (Decadron)	**Rifapentine** (Priftin)
Imipramine (Tofranil)	**Efavirenz** (Sustiva)	**St. John's wort**
Nortriptyline (Aventyl)	**Lumacaftor** (Orkambi)	
Protriptyline (Vivactil)	**Nevirapine** (Viramune)	
Trimipramine (Surmontil)	**Oxcarbazepine** (Trileptal)	

COMMENTS: Enzyme inducers may gradually reduce the serum levels and effect of imipramine, desipramine, amitriptyline, and probably other tricyclic antidepressants (TCA). TCAs differ in their metabolism by CYP450 isozymes; hence, the magnitude of TCAs interaction with enzyme inducers may vary as well.

CLASS 3: ASSESS RISK & TAKE ACTION IF NECESSARY
• *Consider Alternative:* While it would be prudent to use an alternative to the enzyme inducer, suitable alternatives with equivalent therapeutic effects are not available for most enzyme

inducers. One could also consider a non-TCA antidepressant, but many of them may also be susceptible to enzyme induction.

- **Monitor**: Monitor for altered tricyclic antidepressant effect if enzyme inducer is initiated, discontinued, or changed in dosage. Keep in mind that enzyme induction is usually gradual and may take days to weeks for onset and offset, depending on the specific inducer.

OBJECT DRUGS	PRECIPITANT DRUGS
Antidepressants, Tricyclic:	**Antidepressants, Other:**
Amitriptyline (Elavil)	**Bupropion** (Wellbutrin)
Amoxapine (Asendin)	**Duloxetine** (Cymbalta)
Clomipramine (Anafranil)	**Fluoxetine** (Prozac)
Desipramine (Norpramin)	**Fluvoxamine** (Luvox)
Doxepin (Sinequan)	**Nefazodone**
Imipramine (Tofranil)	**Paroxetine** (Paxil)
Nortriptyline (Aventyl)	
Protriptyline (Vivactil)	
Trimipramine (Surmontil)	

COMMENTS: Antidepressants that inhibit CYP2D6 (and to a lesser extent inhibit CYP1A2 and CYP3A4) can increase tricyclic antidepressant (TCA) serum concentrations possibly leading to toxicity (e.g., dry mouth, urinary retention, blurred vision, tachycardia, constipation, and postural hypotension). With most inhibitors, the onset and offset of the interaction occurs over several days to a week, but it may take up to several weeks with fluoxetine. Combinations of TCAs and enzyme inhibitors (e.g., fluoxetine or paroxetine) are sometimes used intentionally to increase antidepressant efficacy.

CLASS 3: ASSESS RISK & TAKE ACTION IF NECESSARY
- **Consider Alternative**:
  Antidepressants, Other: **Sertraline** (Zoloft), **citalopram** (Celexa), **escitalopram** (Lexapro), **desvenlafaxine** (Pristiq), and **venlafaxine** (Effexor) have less effect on CYP2D6 than fluoxetine or paroxetine. Larger than usual doses of desvenlafaxine (eg, 400 mg/day) may produce moderate CYP2D6 inhibition, but little inhibition occurs at 100 mg/day.
- **Monitor**: Monitor for altered TCA response if an SSRI that is an enzyme inhibitor is initiated, discontinued, or changed in dosage.

OBJECT DRUGS	PRECIPITANT DRUGS	
Antidepressants, Tricyclic:	**Enzyme Inhibitors:**	
Amitriptyline (Elavil)	**Abiraterone** (Zytiga)	**Mirabegron** (Myrbetriq)
Amoxapine (Asendin)	**Amiodarone** (Cordarone)	**Propafenone** (Rythmol)
Clomipramine (Anafranil)	**Atazanavir** (Reyataz)	**Propoxyphene***
Desipramine (Norpramin)	**Cimetidine** (Tagamet)	**Quinidine** (Quinidex)
Doxepin (Sinequan)	**Cinacalcet** (Sensipar)	**Ranolazine** (Ranexa)
Imipramine (Tofranil)	**Clobazam** (Onfi)	**Ritonavir** (Norvir)
Nortriptyline (Aventyl)	**Conivaptan** (Vaprisol)	**Terbinafine** (Lamisil)
Protriptyline (Vivactil)	**Diphenhydramine** (Benadryl)	**Thioridazine** (Mellaril)
Trimipramine (Surmontil)	**Haloperidol** (Haldol)	

* Propoxyphene (Darvon) was withdrawn from the US market.

COMMENTS: CYP2D6 inhibitors (and to a lesser extent inhibitors of CYP1A2 and CYP3A4) can increase tricyclic antidepressant (TCA) serum concentrations possibly leading to toxicity (e.g., dry mouth, urinary retention, blurred vision, tachycardia, constipation, and postural hypotension). Both bupropion and tricyclic antidepressants can lower the seizure threshold, so theoretically the combination may increase the risk of seizures. Note that because terbinafine has an extraordinarily long terminal half-life, the inhibitory effect of terbinafine on CYP2D6 may last for many weeks after terbinafine is discontinued.

CLASS 3: ASSESS RISK & TAKE ACTION IF NECESSARY
- **Consider Alternative**:
  Cimetidine: Other acid suppressors are unlikely to interact. Consider using **famotidine** (Pepcid), **nizatidine** (Axid), **ranitidine** (Zantac), **dexlansoprazole** (Kapidex), **esomeprazole** (Nexium), **omeprazole** (Prilosec), **lansoprazole** (Prevacid), **rabeprazole** (Aciphex), or **pantoprazole** (Protonix).
  Diphenhydramine: Nonsedating antihistamines are unlikely to inhibit CYP2D6.
- **Monitor**: Monitor for altered TCA response if an enzyme inhibitor is initiated, discontinued, or changed in dosage.

14

OBJECT DRUGS	PRECIPITANT DRUGS
Antidiabetic Agents:	**Beta-Blockers, Nonselective:**
Alogliptin (Nesina)	**Carteolol** (Ocupress)
Chlorpropamide (Diabinese)	**Carvedilol** (Coreg)
Glimepiride (Amaryl)	**Labetalol** (Trandate)
Glipizide (Glucotrol)	**Levobunolol** (Betagan)
Glyburide (DiaBeta, Glucovance)	**Nadolol** (Corgard)
Insulin	**Penbutolol** (Levatol)
Linagliptin (Tradjenta)	**Pindolol** (Visken)
Metformin (Glucophage)	**Propranolol** (Inderal)
Nateglinide (Starlix)	**Sotalol** (Betapace)
Pioglitazone (Actos)	**Timolol** (Blocadren)
Repaglinide (Prandin)	
Rosiglitazone (Avandia)	
Saxagliptin (Onglyza)	
Tolbutamide (Orinase)	

COMMENTS: Noncardioselective beta-adrenergic blockers may prolong the duration of a hypoglycemic reaction; patients may also develop hypertensive reactions with compensatory bradycardia during hypoglycemia. All beta-blockers inhibit hypoglycemia-induced tachycardia, but sweating is not inhibited.

CLASS 2: USE ONLY IF BENEFIT FELT TO OUTWEIGH RISK
- *Use Alternative*: Avoid nonselective beta-adrenergic blockers in patients receiving antidiabetic agents if possible. If beta-blockers are used, cardioselective agents are preferred, since they are less likely to prolong hypoglycemia or produce hypertensive reactions during hypoglycemia. Cardioselective beta-blockers include **acebutolol** (Sectral), **atenolol** (Tenormin), **betaxolol** (Kerlone), and **metoprolol** (Lopressor).
- *Monitor*: Diabetic patients taking beta-blockers should be warned that hypoglycemic episodes may not result in tachycardia.

OBJECT DRUGS	PRECIPITANT DRUGS
Antidiabetic Agents	**Azole Antifungals:**
(CYP2C9 Substrates):	**Fluconazole** (Diflucan)
Chlorpropamide (Diabinese)	**Miconazole** (Monistat)
Glimepiride (Amaryl)	**Voriconazole** (Vfend)
Glipizide (Glucotrol)	
Glyburide (DiaBeta)	
Nateglinide (Starlix)	
Rosiglitazone (Avandia)	
Tolbutamide (Orinase)	

COMMENTS: Oral hypoglycemic drugs that are metabolized by CYP2C9 may produce enhanced hypoglycemic effects when administered with azole antifungal agents that inhibit the enzyme. Nateglinide and rosiglitazone both have additional pathways of metabolism and may be less affected by inhibitors of only one pathway.

CLASS 3: ASSESS RISK & TAKE ACTION IF NECESSARY
- *Consider Alternative*: Itraconazole (Sporanox) and terbinafine (Lamisil) are antifungals that do not inhibit CYP2C9. Ketoconazole (Nizoral) has been reported to increase the plasma concentrations of rosiglitazone and tolbutamide.
- *Monitor*: Diabetic patients taking CYP2C9-inhibiting antifungals should be warned that hypoglycemic episodes may occur more frequently and should monitor their blood glucose concentrations.

OBJECT DRUGS	PRECIPITANT DRUGS
Antidiabetic Agents:	**Enzyme Inhibitors:**
(CYP2C9 Substrates):	**Amiodarone** (Cordarone)
Chlorpropamide (Diabinese)	**Capecitabine** (Xeloda)
Glimepiride (Amaryl)	**Ceritinib** (Zykadia)
Glipizide (Glucotrol)	**Co-trimoxazole** (Septra)
Glyburide (DiaBeta, Glucovance)	**Delavirdine** (Rescriptor)
Nateglinide (Starlix)	**Efavirenz** (Sustiva)
Rosiglitazone (Avandia)	**Etravirine** (Intelence)
Tolbutamide (Orinase)	**Fluorouracil** (Adrucil)
	Fluoxetine (Prozac)
	Fluvastatin (Lescol)
	Fluvoxamine (Luvox)
	Metronidazole (Flagyl)
	Sulfinpyrazone (Anturane)

COMMENTS: Oral hypoglycemic drugs that are metabolized by CYP2C9 may produce enhanced hypoglycemic effects when administered with a CYP2C9 inhibitor. Nateglinide and rosiglitazone both have additional pathways of metabolism and may be less affected by inhibitors of only one pathway. Co-trimoxazole, however, inhibits two pathways for rosiglitazone metabolism; the trimethoprim component inhibits CYP2C8, and the sulfamethoxazole component inhibits CYP2C9. Single doses of metronidazole would be unlikely to produce hypoglycemia when combined with these antidiabetic agents.

CLASS 3: ASSESS RISK & TAKE ACTION IF NECESSARY
- *Consider Alternative*:
  Fluvastatin: **Atorvastatin** (Lipitor), **lovastatin** (Mevacor), **pravastatin** (Pravachol), **rosuvastatin** (Crestor), and **simvastatin** (Zocor) do not appear to inhibit CYP2C9.
  Fluoxetine / Fluvoxamine: Other SSRI antidepressants would not be expected to interact.
- *Monitor*: Monitor for hypoglycemic episodes during coadministration of CYP2C9 inhibitors.

OBJECT DRUGS	PRECIPITANT DRUGS	
Antidiabetic Agents	**Antimicrobials:**	
(CYP3A4 Substrates):	**Ciprofloxacin** (Cipro)	**Ketoconazole** (Nizoral)
Nateglinide (Starlix)	**Clarithromycin** (Biaxin)	**Posaconazole** (Noxafil)
Pioglitazone (Actos)	**Erythromycin** (E-Mycin)	**Quinupristin** (Synercid)
Repaglinide (Prandin)	**Fluconazole** (Diflucan)	**Telithromycin** (Ketek)
Saxagliptin (Onglyza)	**Isoniazid** (INH)	**Troleandomycin** (TAO)
Sitagliptin (Janumet)	**Itraconazole** (Sporanox)	**Voriconazole** (Vfend)

COMMENTS: Some antimicrobials can reduce oral hypoglycemic metabolism and produce hypoglycemic episodes. Pioglitazone and repaglinide are also metabolized by CYP2C8, and people taking a CYP2C8 inhibitor in addition to a CYP3A4 inhibitor may have large interactions. For example, patients taking repaglinide (a substrate of CYP3A4, CYP2C8, and OATP) with both gemfibrozil (an inhibitor of both CYP2C8 and OATP) and itraconazole (CYP3A4 inhibitor) may have 20-fold increases in repaglinide plasma concentrations. (See CYP Table at front of book for other CYP2C8 and OATP inhibitors.)

CLASS 3: ASSESS RISK & TAKE ACTION IF NECESSARY
- *Consider Alternative*:
  Azole Antifungals: Fluconazole appears to be a less potent inhibitor of CYP3A4; but in larger doses it also inhibits CYP3A4. **Terbinafine** (Lamisil) does not appear to affect CYP3A4.
  Macrolide Antibiotics: **Azithromycin** (Zithromax) and **dirithromycin*** do not appear to inhibit CYP3A4 and are unlikely to interact. (*not available in US)
  Telithromycin: The use of **azithromycin** (Zithromax) or a quinolone antibiotic other than ciprofloxacin should be considered.
- *Monitor*: Monitor for hypoglycemic episodes during azole antifungal or macrolide coadministration.

OBJECT DRUGS	PRECIPITANT DRUGS
Antidiabetic Agents (CYP3A4 Substrates): Nateglinide (Starlix) Pioglitazone (Actos) Repaglinide (Prandin) Saxagliptin (Onglyza) Sitagliptin (Janumet)	**Calcium Channel Blockers:** Diltiazem (Cardizem) Verapamil (Isoptin)

COMMENTS: Diltiazem and verapamil (both are CYP3A4 inhibitors) could reduce oral hypoglycemic metabolism and produce hypoglycemic episodes. Pioglitazone and repaglinide are also metabolized by CYP2C8, and people taking a CYP2C8 inhibitor in addition to a CYP3A4 inhibitor may have large interactions. For example, patients taking repaglinide with both gemfibrozil (CYP2C8 inhibitor) and itraconazole (CYP3A4 inhibitor) may have 20-fold increases in repaglinide plasma concentrations. (See CYP Table at front of book for other CYP2C8 inhibitors.)

CLASS 3: ASSESS RISK & TAKE ACTION IF NECESSARY
* *Consider Alternative:*
  Calcium channel blockers: Agents other than diltiazem and verapamil are unlikely to inhibit the metabolism of these antidiabetic agents.
* *Monitor:* Monitor for hypoglycemic episodes during calcium channel blocker coadministration.

OBJECT DRUGS	PRECIPITANT DRUGS	
Antidiabetic Agents **CYP3A4 Substrates):** Nateglinide (Starlix) Pioglitazone (Actos) Repaglinide (Prandin) Saxagliptin (Onglyza) Sitagliptin (Janumet)	**Enzyme Inhibitors:** Amiodarone (Cordarone) Amprenavir (Agenerase) Aprepitant (Emend) Atazanavir (Reyataz) Boceprevir (Victrelis) Ceritinib (Zykadia) Cobicistat (Stribild) Conivaptan (Vaprisol) Cyclosporine (Neoral) Darunavir (Prezista) Delavirdine (Rescriptor)	Fluvoxamine (Luvox) Grapefruit Indinavir (Crixivan) Lomitapide (Juxtapid) Mifepristone (Korlym) Nefazodone Nelfinavir (Viracept) Ritonavir (Norvir) Saquinavir (Invirase) Telaprevir (Incivek)

COMMENTS: Although data are limited, any CYP3A4 inhibitor could reduce oral hypoglycemic metabolism and produce hypoglycemic episodes. Pioglitazone and repaglinide are also metabolized by CYP2C8, and people taking a CYP2C8 inhibitor in addition to a CYP3A4 inhibitor may have large interactions. For example, patients taking repaglinide with both gemfibrozil (CYP2C8 inhibitor) and itraconazole (CYP3A4 inhibitor) may have 20-fold increases in repaglinide plasma concentrations. (See CYP Table at front of book for other CYP2C8 inhibitors.)

CLASS 3: ASSESS RISK & TAKE ACTION IF NECESSARY
* *Consider Alternative:*
  Antidepressants: **Sertraline** (Zoloft), **citalopram** (Celexa), **escitalopram** (Lexapro), **desvenlafaxine** (Pristiq), **venlafaxine** (Effexor), and **paroxetine** (Paxil) appear less likely to inhibit CYP3A4 than fluvoxamine. **Fluoxetine** (Prozac) appears to be a weak inhibitor of CYP3A4.
  Grapefruit: Orange juice does not appear to inhibit CYP3A4.
* *Circumvent/Minimize:* In one study, giving repaglinide either 1 hour before or 3 hours after cyclosporine minimized the increase in repaglinide concentrations. It is not known if separating doses would circumvent the interactions of other combinations listed above.
* *Monitor:* Monitor for hypoglycemic episodes during the coadministration of CYP3A4 inhibitors.

OBJECT DRUGS	PRECIPITANT DRUGS
Antidiabetic Agents (CYP2C8 Substrates):	**Clopidogrel** (Plavix)
Pioglitazone (Actos)	**Deferasirox** (Exjade)
Repaglinide (Prandin)	**Gemfibrozil** (Lopid)
Rosiglitazone (Avandia)	**Lapatinib** (Tykerb)

COMMENTS: Gemfibrozil markedly increases plasma concentrations of repaglinide, probably through gemfibrozil-induced inhibition of CYP2C8 and probably UGT (the role of OATP1B1 is under investigation). Clopidogrel and deferasirox inhibit CYP2C8 and have also been shown to increase plasma concentrations of repaglinide about 5-fold and 2-fold respectively. Lapatinib is also a CYP2C8 inhibitor, and is likely to interact with these antidiabetic agents. These combination would be expected to increase the risk of hypoglycemia. The inhibitory effect of gemfibrozil on repaglinide metabolism appears to last at least 12 hours, well after the gemfibrozil is largely eliminated. When a potent CYP3A4 inhibitor (itraconazole) was given in addition to gemfibrozil, plasma concentrations of repaglinide were increased almost 20-fold.

CLASS 2: USE ONLY IF BENEFIT FELT TO OUTWEIGH RISK
- *Use Alternative:* It would be prudent to use an alternative to one of the drugs.
  Gemfibrozil: Little is known about the effect of fibrates other than gemfibrozil on repaglinide pharmacokinetics. In vitro studies suggest that **fenofibrate** (Tricor) may also inhibit the CYP2C8 metabolism of repaglinide, but perhaps to a lesser degree.
  Repaglinide: Study in healthy subjects suggests that gemfibrozil has little effect on **nateglinide** (Starlix) metabolism. Gemfibrozil would be expected to have little or no effect on many other antidiabetics given that most of them are metabolized primarily by enzymes other than CYP2C8.
- *Circumvent/Minimize:* Consider using conservative doses of repaglinide if it is used concurrently with gemfibrozil.
- *Monitor:* In patients receiving repaglinide, monitor blood glucose carefully if gemfibrozil is started, stopped, or changed in dosage.

OBJECT DRUGS	PRECIPITANT DRUGS	
Antidiabetic Agents:	**Gastric Alkalinizers:**	
Glipizide (Glucotrol)	**Antacids**	**Nizatidine** (Axid)
Glyburide (DiaBeta,	**Cimetidine** (Tagamet)	**Omeprazole** (Prilosec)
Glucovance)	**Dexlansoprazole** (Kapidex)	**Pantoprazole** (Protonix)
	Esomeprazole (Nexium)	**Rabeprazole** (Aciphex)
	Famotidine (Pepcid)	**Ranitidine** (Zantac)
	Lansoprazole (Prevacid)	

COMMENTS: Antacids have been reported to increase the rate or amount of absorption of glipizide and glyburide and to increase their hypoglycemic effects. Ranitidine was reported to increase the hypoglycemic effects of glipizide. If these effects are due to changes in gastric pH, other gastric alkalinizers would likely have a similar effect.

CLASS 3: ASSESS RISK & TAKE ACTION IF NECESSARY
- *Circumvent/Minimize:* Administration of the glipizide or glyburide two hours before an antacid would avoid the interactions. It may be difficult to separate the doses of an H_2-antagonist or PPI to ensure no interaction occurs.
- *Consider Alternative:* Other oral hypoglycemic agents such as **chlorpropamide** (Diabinese), **metformin** (Glucophage), **tolbutamide** (Orinase), or **rosiglitazone** (Avandia) may avoid interactions with gastric alkalinizers.
- *Monitor:* The administration of gastric alkalinizers to patients taking glipizide or glyburide should be accompanied by careful blood glucose monitoring.

OBJECT DRUGS	PRECIPITANT DRUGS	
Antihypertensive Drugs:	**NSAIDs:**	
ACE Inhibitors (ACEIs)	**Aspirin**	**Meclofenamate**
Angiotensin Receptor Blockers	**Diclofenac** (Voltaren)	**Mefenamic acid**
(ARBs)	**Diflunisal** (Dolobid)	**Meloxicam** (Mobic)
	Etodolac (Lodine)	**Nabumetone** (Relafen)
	Fenoprofen (Nalfon)	**Naproxen** (Aleve)
	Flurbiprofen (Ansaid)	**Oxaprozin** (Daypro)
	Ibuprofen (Motrin)	**Piroxicam** (Feldene)
	Indomethacin (Indocin)	**Sulindac** (Clinoril)
	Ketoprofen (Orudis)	**Tolmetin** (Tolectin)
	Ketorolac (Toradol)	

COMMENTS: In patients receiving ACEIs or ARBs for hypertension concurrent use of NSAIDs can substantially reduce the antihypertensive response. In most cases the effect is gradual, so short-term use of NSAIDs (i.e., a few days) in patients with well-controlled hypertension is unlikely to cause problems. Low-dose aspirin does not appear to have much effect on antihypertensive therapy. NSAIDs may also interfere with the efficacy of ACEIs, ARBs and diuretics used in the treatment of heart failure.

CLASS 3: ASSESS RISK & TAKE ACTION IF NECESSARY
* *Consider Alternative*:

NSAID: If possible use a non-NSAID analgesic such as acetaminophen. If a NSAID is required, use the lowest effective dose. There is some evidence to suggest that certain NSAIDs may have less effect than others on blood pressure, so if one NSAID is a problem, consider trying a different NSAID. It is not established that COX-2 inhibitors such as **celecoxib** (Celebrex) avoid the interaction but they could be tried. Because non-acetylated salicylates such as **choline magnesium trisalicylate** (Trilisate), **magnesium salicylates**, and **salsalate** (Disalcid) have less effect on prostaglandins than aspirin, they may be less likely to interact.

Antihypertensive: Although ACEIs and ARBs appear to be particularly susceptible to interactions with NSAIDs, diuretics and other antihypertensives may be affected as well. Nonetheless, in cases where it is not possible to modify the NSAID therapy, it may be possible to control the hypertension by using antihypertensive agents other than ACEIs or ARBs. Some recommend the use of calcium channel blockers if NSAIDs are preventing antihypertensive control.
* *Monitor*: If NSAIDs are used in patients on antihypertensive therapy, monitor the blood pressure carefully. Keep in mind that the effect may take place gradually over 2 to 3 weeks after starting the NSAID. Blood pressure monitoring is also warranted if the NSAID dose is changed or discontinued, or if the patient is switched from one NSAID to another.

OBJECT DRUGS	PRECIPITANT DRUGS
Antimetabolites:	**Allopurinol** (Zyloprim)
Azathioprine (Imuran)	**Febuxostat** (Uloric)
Mercaptopurine (Purinethol)	

COMMENTS: Allopurinol and febuxostat inhibit the metabolism of mercaptopurine, which is also the active metabolite of azathioprine. This effect considerably increases antimetabolite effect and toxicity of both azathioprine and mercaptopurine. Generally, these combinations should be avoided, but they have sometimes been used intentionally with careful monitoring. For example, several studies in patients with inflammatory bowel disease suggest that low dose allopurinol (with lowered azathioprine dose and careful monitoring) may improve azathioprine efficacy without increasing toxicity. This may also be true when azathioprine or mercaptopurine is used to treat other diseases.

CLASS 2: USE ONLY IF BENEFIT FELT TO OUTWEIGH RISK
- *Use Alternative:* Patients taking azathioprine or mercaptopurine should generally not be administered allopurinol or febuxostat unless it is being done intentionally to improve efficacy.
- *Circumvent/Minimize:* If allopurinol is added to azathioprine or mercaptopurine therapy, it is generally recommended that the azathioprine or mercaptopurine dose be reduced to 25% to 33% of the original dose. Lower than normal doses of allopurinol have also been suggested.
- *Monitor:* If the combination is used, monitor for evidence of bone marrow suppression, and instruct the patient to contact their prescriber immediately if they experience evidence of pancytopenia such as fever, sore throat, easy bruising, or bleeding.

OBJECT DRUGS	PRECIPITANT DRUGS
Antimetabolites:	**Ribavirin** (Rebetol)
Azathioprine (Imuran)	
Mercaptopurine (Purinethol)	

COMMENTS: Ribavirin appears to inhibit one of the steps in the metabolism of azathioprine and mercaptopurine, and may increase the risk of toxicity, usually bone marrow suppression. A number of patients have developed severe pancytopenia, usually after several weeks of combined therapy.

CLASS 2: USE ONLY IF BENEFIT FELT TO OUTWEIGH RISK
- *Circumvent/Minimize:* If appropriate for the patient, it may be prudent to withdraw azathioprine or mercaptopurine therapy during ribavirin therapy. If the combination is used, it may be necessary to reduce the dose of azathioprine or mercaptopurine.
- *Monitor:* If the combination is used, monitor for evidence of bone marrow suppression, and instruct the patient to contact their prescriber immediately if they experience evidence of pancytopenia such as fever, sore throat, easy bruising, or bleeding.

OBJECT DRUGS	PRECIPITANT DRUGS	
Antipsychotics, Atypical:	**Enzyme Inducers:**	
Aripiprazole (Abilify)	**Barbiturates**	**Phenytoin** (Dilantin)
Brexpiprazole (Rexulti)	**Bosentan** (Tracleer)	**Primidone** (Mysoline)
Clozapine (Clozaril)	**Carbamazepine** (Tegretol)	**Rifabutin** (Mycobutin)
Iloperidone (Fanapt)	**Dabrafenib** (Tafinlar)	**Rifampin** (Rifadin)
Lurasidone (Latuda)	**Dexamethasone** (Decadron)	**Rifapentine** (Priftin)
Olanzapine (Zyprexa)	**Efavirenz** (Sustiva)	**St. John's wort**
Quetiapine (Seroquel)	**Lumacaftor** (Orkambi)	
Risperidone (Risperdal)	**Nevirapine** (Viramune)	
Ziprasidone (Geodon)	**Oxcarbazepine** (Trileptal)	

COMMENTS: These antipsychotics are metabolized by CYP3A4; drugs that induce CYP3A4 may reduce their serum levels resulting in loss of efficacy. For example, carbamazepine may reduce olanzapine concentrations by about 50%.

CLASS 3: ASSESS RISK & TAKE ACTION IF NECESSARY
- *Consider Alternative:* Use an alternative to the enzyme inducer if possible. **Paliperidone** (Invega) is not metabolized by CYP3A4 and could be considered as an alternative.
- *Circumvent/Minimize:* The manufacturer recommends that the dose of aripiprazole be doubled (to 20-30 mg/day) if CYP3A4 inducers are added. If the enzyme inducer is then discontinued, they recommend that the aripiprazole dose be decreased to 10-15 mg/day.
- *Monitor:* If it is necessary to use an antipsychotic and enzyme inducer, monitor for altered antipsychotic effect if an enzyme inducer is started, stopped, or changed in dosage. Keep in mind that enzyme induction is usually gradual and may take days to weeks for onset and offset, depending on the specific inducer.

OBJECT DRUGS	PRECIPITANT DRUGS
Antipsychotics, Atypical:	**Antimicrobials:**
Aripiprazole (Abilify)	**Ciprofloxacin** (Cipro)
Brexpiprazole (Rexulti)	**Clarithromycin** (Biaxin)
Clozapine (Clozaril)	**Erythromycin** (E-Mycin)
Iloperidone (Fanapt)	**Fluconazole** (Diflucan)
Lurasidone (Latuda)	**Itraconazole** (Sporanox)
Olanzapine (Zyprexa)	**Ketoconazole** (Nizoral)
Quetiapine (Seroquel)	**Posaconazole** (Noxafil)
Risperidone (Risperdal)	**Quinupristin** (Synercid)
Ziprasidone (Geodon)	**Telithromycin** (Ketek)
	Troleandomycin (TAO)
	Voriconazole (Vfend)

COMMENTS: These antipsychotics are metabolized by CYP3A4; these antimicrobials inhibit CYP3A4, and may increase antipsychotic serum levels.

CLASS 3: ASSESS RISK & TAKE ACTION IF NECESSARY
- *Consider Alternative*:
  Azole Antifungals: Itraconazole and ketoconazole are potent inhibitors of CYP3A4; fluconazole appears weaker, but in larger doses it also inhibits CYP3A4.
  Macrolides: Unlike erythromycin, clarithromycin and troleandomycin, **azithromycin** (Zithromax) and **dirithromycin*** do not appear to inhibit CYP3A4. (*not available in US) Telithromycin: The use of **azithromycin** (Zithromax) or a quinolone antibiotic other than ciprofloxacin may be considered.
  Paliperidone (Invega) is not metabolized by CYP3A4 and could be considered as an alternative.
- *Circumvent/Minimize*: The manufacturer recommends that the dose of aripiprazole be reduced to one-half the usual dose if CYP3A4 inhibitors are added. If the CYP3A4 inhibitor is then discontinued, they recommend that the aripiprazole dose be increased to the usual dosage.
- *Monitor*: Be alert for altered effect of the antipsychotic if CYP3A4 inhibitors are started, stopped, or changed in dosage. Due to the long half-lives of some of these drugs, the onset and offset of these interactions may take 1-2 weeks.

OBJECT DRUGS	PRECIPITANT DRUGS
Antipsychotics, Atypical:	**Antidepressants:**
Aripiprazole (Abilify)	**Bupropion** (Wellbutrin)
Brexpiprazole (Rexulti)	**Duloxetine** (Cymbalta)
Clozapine (Clozaril)	**Fluoxetine** (Prozac)
Iloperidone (Fanapt)	**Fluvoxamine** (Luvox)
Olanzapine (Zyprexa)	**Paroxetine** (Paxil)
Paliperidone (Invega)	
Risperidone (Risperdal)	

COMMENTS: These antipsychotics are metabolized by CYP2D6. These antidepressants inhibit CYP2D6 and may lead to accumulation of the antipsychotics.

CLASS 3: ASSESS RISK & TAKE ACTION IF NECESSARY
- *Consider Alternative*: Antidepressants with small or no effects on CYP2D6 include **citalopram** (Celexa), **escitalopram** (Lexapro), **venlafaxine** (Effexor), **desvenlafaxine** (Pristiq), and **sertraline** (Zoloft).
- *Circumvent/Minimize*: The manufacturer recommends that the dose of aripiprazole be reduced to one-half the usual dose if CYP2D6 inhibitors are added. If the inhibitor is then discontinued, they recommend that the aripiprazole dose be increased to the usual dosage.
- *Monitor*: Be alert for altered effect of the antipsychotics if CYP2D6 inhibitors are started, stopped, or changed in dosage. Due to the long half-lives of some of these drugs, the onset and offset of these interactions may take 1-2 weeks.

OBJECT DRUGS	PRECIPITANT DRUGS	
Antipsychotics, Atypical:	**Enzyme Inhibitors: (CYP3A4)**	
Aripiprazole (Abilify)	**Amiodarone** (Cordarone)	**Diltiazem** (Cardizem)
Brexpiprazole (Rexulti)	**Amprenavir** (Agenerase)	**Grapefruit**
Clozapine (Clozaril)	**Aprepitant** (Emend)	**Indinavir** (Crixivan)
Iloperidone (Fanapt)	**Atazanavir** (Reyataz)	**Lomitapide** (Juxtapid)
Lurasidone (Latuda)	**Boceprevir** (Victrelis)	**Mifepristone** (Korlym)
Olanzapine (Zyprexa)	**Ceritinib** (Zykadia)	**Nefazodone**
Quetiapine (Seroquel)	**Cobicistat** (Stribild)	**Nelfinavir** (Viracept)
Risperidone (Risperdal)	**Conivaptan** (Vaprisol)	**Ritonavir** (Norvir)
Ziprasidone (Geodon)	**Cyclosporine** (Neoral)	**Saquinavir** (Invirase)
	Darunavir (Prezista)	**Telaprevir** (Incivek)
	Delavirdine (Rescriptor)	**Verapamil** (Isoptin)

COMMENTS: These antipsychotics are metabolized by CYP3A4; drugs that inhibit CYP3A4 may increase antipsychotic serum levels. Most of these antipsychotics have multiple pathways of elimination (see CYP2D6 inhibitors, below), and the magnitude of the interactions is likely to vary substantially depending on the specific pair of drugs, and the specific patient characteristics.

CLASS 3: ASSESS RISK & TAKE ACTION IF NECESSARY
- *Consider Alternative*: Use an alternative to the enzyme inhibitor if possible.
  Calcium channel blockers: Calcium channel blockers other than diltiazem and verapamil are unlikely to inhibit CYP3A4.
  Grapefruit: Orange juice does not appear to inhibit CYP3A4.
  Antipsychotic: **Paliperidone** (Invega) is not metabolized by CYP3A4 and could be considered as an alternative.
- *Circumvent/Minimize*: The manufacturer recommends that the dose of aripiprazole or be reduced to one-half the usual dose if CYP3A4 inhibitors or CYP2D6 inhibitors are added. If the inhibitor is then discontinued, they recommend that the aripiprazole dose be increased to the usual dosage.
- *Monitor*: Be alert for altered effect of the antipsychotic if CYP3A4 inhibitors are started, stopped, or changed in dosage.

OBJECT DRUGS	PRECIPITANT DRUGS	
Antipsychotics, Atypical:	**Enzyme Inhibitors: (CYP2D6)**	
Aripiprazole (Abilify)	**Abiraterone** (Zytiga)	**Propafenone** (Rythmol)
Brexpiprazole (Rexulti)	**Amiodarone** (Cordarone)	**Propoxyphene***
Clozapine (Clozaril)	**Cinacalcet** (Sensipar)	**Quinidine** (Quinidex)
Iloperidone (Fanapt)	**Clobazam** (Onfi)	**Ritonavir** (Norvir)
Olanzapine (Zyprexa)	**Diphenhydramine** (Benadryl)	**Terbinafine** (Lamisil)
Paliperidone (Invega)	**Haloperidol** (Haldol)	**Thioridazine** (Mellaril)
Perphenazine (Trilafon)	**Mirabegron** (Myrbetriq)	
Risperidone (Risperdal)		

* Propoxyphene (Darvon) was withdrawn from the US market.

COMMENTS: These antipsychotics are metabolized by CYP2D6. Drugs that inhibit CYP2D6 may lead to accumulation of the antipsychotic. People with "normal" CYP2D6 activity (Extensive Metabolizers) are at the greatest risk. Most of these antipsychotics have multiple pathways of elimination (see CYP3A4 inhibitors, above), and the magnitude of the interactions is likely to vary substantially depending on the specific pair of drugs, and the specific patient characteristics. Note that because terbinafine has an extraordinarily long terminal half-life, the inhibitory effect of terbinafine on CYP2D6 may last for many weeks after terbinafine is discontinued. In one case perphenazine toxicity (akathisia) persisted for 3 weeks after stopping terbinafine. (Perphenazine is not technically an "atypical" antipsychotic.)

CLASS 3: ASSESS RISK & TAKE ACTION IF NECESSARY
- *Consider Alternative*:
  Diphenhydramine: Other antihistamines such as **desloratadine** (Clarinex), **fexofenadine** (Allegra), **loratadine** Claritin), and **cetirizine** (Zyrtec) are not known to inhibit CYP2D6.
- *Monitor*: Be alert for altered effect of these antipsychotics if CYP2D6 inhibitors are started, stopped, or changed in dosage. The iloperidone product information suggests lowering the iloperidone dose by 50% when it is used with CYP2D6 inhibitors. Due to the long half-lives of some of these drugs, the onset and offset of these interactions may take one to two weeks.

OBJECT DRUGS	PRECIPITANT DRUGS	
Antipsychotics, Atypical:	**Enzyme Inhibitors:**	
Asenapine (Saphris)	**Atazanavir** (Reyataz)	**Enoxacin** (Penetrex)
Clozapine (Clozaril)	**Caffeine**	**Mexiletine** (Mexitil)
Olanzapine (Zyprexa)	**Cimetidine** (Tagamet)	**Tacrine** (Cognex)
	Ciprofloxacin (Cipro)	**Zileuton** (Zyflo)
	Contraceptives, Oral	

COMMENTS: Agents that inhibit CYP1A2 and possibly CYP2C19 increase antipsychotic plasma levels. **Enoxacin** is a potent inhibitor of CYP1A2 and would be expected to markedly increase antipsychotic plasma concentrations; it should be considered a **Class 2** interaction. Oral contraceptives are generally modest inhibitors of CYP1A2, and the degree of inhibition is likely to be highly variable depending on the dose of the contraceptive and specific patient characteristics. The ability of caffeine to increase clozapine concentrations has usually been observed after moderate to heavy caffeine use.

CLASS 3: ASSESS RISK & TAKE ACTION IF NECESSARY
- *Consider Alternative*:
  Cimetidine: **Famotidine** (Pepcid), **nizatidine** (Axid), and **ranitidine** (Zantac) have minimal effects on drug metabolism.
  Ciprofloxacin or Enoxacin: **Gemifloxacin** (Factive), **levofloxacin** (Levaquin), **lomefloxacin** (Maxaquin), **moxifloxacin** (Avelox), and **ofloxacin** (Floxin), appear to have little effect on CYP1A2.
- *Monitor*: Monitor for altered antipsychotic response if a CYP1A2 inhibitor is initiated, discontinued, or dose is changed.

OBJECT DRUGS	PRECIPITANT DRUGS
Antipsychotics:	**Fluvoxamine** (Luvox)
Asenapine (Saphris)	
Clozapine (Clozaril)	
Olanzapine (Zyprexa)	

COMMENTS: Agents that inhibit CYP1A2 and possibly CYP2C19 increase antipsychotic plasma levels. Fluvoxamine has a marked effect, and can increase serum clozapine concentrations up to 5-10 fold. Fluvoxamine has been used to increase clozapine efficacy in patients with resistant schizophrenia, but careful monitoring is necessary to avoid clozapine toxicity. Some other SSRIs may produce modest increases in clozapine plasma concentrations, including **fluoxetine**, **paroxetine** and **sertraline**.

CLASS 2: USE ONLY IF BENEFIT FELT TO OUTWEIGH RISK
- *Use Alternative*: Fluoxetine (Prozac), **paroxetine** (Paxil), and **sertraline** (Zoloft) appear to interact less than fluvoxamine. Theoretically, **venlafaxine** (Effexor) would be even less likely to interact, but information is lacking.
- *Monitor*: Monitor for altered antipsychotic response if a CYP1A2 inhibitor such as fluvoxamine is initiated, discontinued, or dose is changed.

OBJECT DRUGS	PRECIPITANT DRUGS
Antipsychotics:	**Smoking Cessation Drugs:**
Clozapine (Clozaril)	**Bupropion** (Zyban)
Olanzapine (Zyprexa)	**Nicotine** (Nicorette, Nicoderm, Nicotrol)
	Varenicline (Chantix)

COMMENTS: Patients on clozapine or olanzapine who stop smoking may develop substantial increases in plasma concentrations of the antipsychotic because smoking markedly enhances the activity of CYP1A2 (important in the metabolism of clozapine and olanzapine). The magnitude of the increase in clozapine or olanzapine levels is highly variable, with some people manifesting dramatic increases and some others developing only small effects.

CLASS 3: ASSESS RISK & TAKE ACTION IF NECESSARY
- *Monitor:* In a patient on clozapine or olanzapine the addition of a smoking cessation drug should be a signal to monitor for evidence of antipsychotic toxicity. Reduce clozapine or olanzapine dose as necessary.

OBJECT DRUGS	PRECIPITANT DRUGS
Antivirals:	**Enzyme Inducers:**
Amprenavir (Agenerase)	**Barbiturates**
Atazanavir (Reyataz)	**Bosentan** (Tracleer)
Daclatasvir (Daklinza)	**Carbamazepine** (Tegretol)
Darunavir (Prezista)	**Dabrafenib** (Tafinlar)
Delavirdine (Rescriptor)	**Dexamethasone** (Decadron)
Etravirine (Intelence)	**Efavirenz** (Sustiva)
Fosamprenavir (Lexiva)	**Etravirine** (Intelence)
Indinavir (Crixivan)	**Lumacaftor** (Orkambi)
Lopinavir (Kaletra)	**Nevirapine** (Viramune)
Maraviroc (Selzentry)	**Oxcarbazepine** (Trileptal)
Nelfinavir (Viracept)	**Phenytoin** (Dilantin)
Rilpivirine (Edurant)	**Primidone** (Mysoline)
Ritonavir (Norvir)	**Rifabutin** (Mycobutin)
Saquinavir (Invirase)	**Rifampin** (Rifadin)
Tipranavir (Aptivus)	**Rifapentine** (Priftin)
	St. John's wort

COMMENTS: Enzyme inducers may reduce the serum levels of the antiviral resulting in loss of efficacy or emergence of resistant viral strains. Some combinations result in dramatic reductions in antiviral serum concentrations (e.g., delavirdine + rifampin, atazanavir + rifampin, and ritonavir + carbamazepine). The combination of ritonavir and rifabutin may increase the risk of rifabutin uveitis (See Rifabutin + Enzyme Inhibitors).

- CLASS 2: USE ONLY IF BENEFIT FELT TO OUTWEIGH RISK
- *Use Alternative:* Use an alternative to the enzyme inducer if possible. Rifampin is particularly problematic, since it can produce dramatic reductions in the plasma concentrations of antivirals.
- *Circumvent/Minimize:* Consider increasing the dose of the antiviral.
- *Monitor:* If it is necessary to use protease inhibitors and enzyme inducers monitor for loss of anti-viral efficacy. Enzyme induction is usually gradual and may take days to weeks for onset and offset, depending on the inducer.

OBJECT DRUGS		PRECIPITANT DRUGS
Antivirals:		**Antimicrobials:**
Amprenavir (Agenerase)	**Lopinavir** (Kaletra)	**Ciprofloxacin** (Cipro)
Atazanavir (Reyataz)	**Maraviroc** (Selzentry)	**Clarithromycin** (Biaxin)
Daclatasvir (Daklinza)	**Nelfinavir** (Viracept)	**Erythromycin** (E-Mycin)
Darunavir (Prezista)	**Rilpivirine** (Edurant)	**Fluconazole** (Diflucan)
Delavirdine (Rescriptor)	**Ritonavir** (Norvir)	**Itraconazole** (Sporanox)
Etravirine (Intelence)	**Saquinavir** (Invirase)	**Ketoconazole** (Nizoral)
Fosamprenavir (Lexiva)	**Tipranavir** (Aptivus)	**Posaconazole** (Noxafil)
Indinavir (Crixivan)		**Quinupristin** (Synercid)
		Telithromycin (Ketek)
		Troleandomycin (TAO)
		Voriconazole (Vfend)

COMMENTS: Inhibitors of CYP3A4 may increase the serum levels of the antivirals resulting in increased side effects. **Ritonavir** may substantially increase **voriconazole** plasma concentrations, especially in patients deficient in CYP2C19.

CLASS 3: ASSESS RISK & TAKE ACTION IF NECESSARY
- *Consider Alternative*:
  Azole Antifungals: Itraconazole and ketoconazole are potent inhibitors of CYP3A4; fluconazole appears weaker, but in larger doses it also inhibits CYP3A4. **Terbinafine** (Lamisil) does not appear to affect CYP3A4, and would not be expected to interact with these antivirals.
  Macrolide Antibiotics: Unlike erythromycin, clarithromycin and troleandomycin, **azithromycin** (Zithromax) and **dirithromycin*** do not appear to inhibit CYP3A4. (*not available in US)
  Telithromycin: The use of **azithromycin** (Zithromax) or a quinolone antibiotic other than ciprofloxacin should be considered.
- *Circumvent/Minimize*: Consider reducing the dose of the antiviral if enzyme inhibitors are coadministered.
- *Monitor*: Monitor for antiviral toxicity.

OBJECT DRUGS		PRECIPITANT DRUGS
Antivirals:		**Antidepressants:**
Amprenavir (Agenerase)	**Lopinavir** (Kaletra)	**Fluvoxamine** (Luvox)
Atazanavir (Reyataz)	**Maraviroc** (Selzentry)	**Nefazodone**
Daclatasvir (Daklinza)	**Nelfinavir** (Viracept)	
Darunavir (Prezista)	**Rilpivirine** (Edurant)	
Delavirdine (Rescriptor)	**Ritonavir** (Norvir)	
Etravirine (Intelence)	**Saquinavir** (Invirase)	
Fosamprenavir (Lexiva)	**Tipranavir** (Aptivus)	
Indinavir (Crixivan)		

COMMENTS: Inhibitors of CYP3A4 may increase the serum levels of these antivirals resulting in increased side effects.

CLASS 3: ASSESS RISK & TAKE ACTION IF NECESSARY
- *Consider Alternative*: Sertraline (Zoloft), **citalopram** (Celexa), **escitalopram** (Lexapro), **venlafaxine** (Effexor), and **paroxetine** (Paxil) appear less likely to inhibit CYP3A4 than fluvoxamine. **Fluoxetine** (Prozac) appears to be a weak inhibitor of CYP3A4, but little is known about the effect of other antidepressants on antivirals.
- *Circumvent/Minimize*: Consider reducing the dose of the antiviral if enzyme inhibitors are coadministered.
- *Monitor*: Monitor for antiviral toxicity.

OBJECT DRUGS	PRECIPITANT DRUGS	
Antivirals:	**Enzyme Inhibitors:**	
Amprenavir (Agenerase)	Amiodarone (Cordarone)	Dronedarone (Multaq)
Atazanavir (Reyataz)	Amprenavir (Agenerase)	Grapefruit
Daclatasvir (Daklinza)	Aprepitant (Emend)	Indinavir (Crixivan)
Darunavir (Prezista)	Atazanavir (Reyataz)	Lomitapide (Juxtapid)
Delavirdine (Rescriptor)	Boceprevir (Victrelis)	Mifepristone (Korlym)
Etravirine (Intelence)	Ceritinib (Zykadia)	Nelfinavir (Viracept)
Fosamprenavir (Lexiva)	Cobicistat (Stribild)	Ritonavir (Norvir)
Indinavir (Crixivan)	Conivaptan (Vaprisol)	Saquinavir (Invirase)
Lopinavir (Kaletra)	Cyclosporine (Neoral)	Telaprevir (Incivek)
Maraviroc (Selzentry)	Darunavir (Prezista)	Verapamil (Isoptin)
Nelfinavir (Viracept)	Delavirdine (Rescriptor)	
Rilpivirine (Edurant)	Diltiazem (Cardizem)	
Ritonavir (Norvir)		
Saquinavir (Invirase)		
Tipranavir (Aptivus)		

COMMENTS: Inhibitors of CYP3A4 may increase the serum levels of the antiviral resulting in increased side effects.

CLASS 3: ASSESS RISK & TAKE ACTION IF NECESSARY
- **Consider Alternative:** Use an alternative to the enzyme inhibitor if possible.
  Calcium channel blockers: Calcium channel blockers other than diltiazem and verapamil are unlikely to inhibit CYP3A4.
  Grapefruit: Orange juice does not appear to inhibit CYP3A4.
- **Circumvent/Minimize:** Consider reducing the dose of the antiviral if enzyme inhibitors are coadministered.
- **Monitor:** Monitor for antiviral toxicity.

OBJECT DRUGS	PRECIPITANT DRUGS	
Antivirals:	**Gastric Antisecretory Agents:**	
Atazanavir (Reyataz)	Cimetidine (Tagamet)	Nizatidine (Axid)
Fosamprenavir (Lexiva)	Dexlansoprazole (Kapidex)	Omeprazole (Prilosec)
Indinavir (Crixivan)	Esomeprazole (Nexium)	Pantoprazole (Protonix)
Nelfinavir (Viracept)	Famotidine (Pepcid)	Rabeprazole (Aciphex)
Rilpivirine (Edurant)	Lansoprazole (Prevacid)	Ranitidine (Zantac)

COMMENTS: Clinical reports suggest that the absorption of some antivirals (especially atazanavir and nelfinavir) may to be reduced by gastric antisecretory agents or antacids.

CLASS 3: ASSESS RISK & TAKE ACTION IF NECESSARY
- **Consider Alternative:** Consider **amprenavir** (Agenerase), **darunavir** (Prezista), **lopinavir** (Kaletra), **ritonavir** (Norvir), or **saquinavir** (Invirase) as alternatives that are minimally affected by elevated gastric pH.
- **Circumvent/Minimize:** Low doses of the gastric antisecretory agent tend to minimize the reduction of antiviral absorption. Separation of the doses of the antiviral from the antisecretory agent or antacid may reduce the magnitude of the interaction.
- **Monitor:** Monitor for reduced antiviral effect in patients treated with a gastric alkalinizer or antacid; adjust dose of protease inhibitor as needed.

OBJECT DRUGS		PRECIPITANT DRUGS
Anxiolytics/Hypnotics		**Antidepressants:**
(CYP3A4 substrates):	**Flurazepam** (Dalmane)	**Fluvoxamine** (Luvox)
Alprazolam (Xanax)	**Halazepam** (Paxipam)	**Nefazodone**
Buspirone (BuSpar)	**Midazolam** (Versed)	
Clonazepam (Klonopin)	**Prazepam** (Centrex)	
Clorazepate (Tranxene)	**Quazepam** (Doral)	
Diazepam (Valium)	**Triazolam** (Halcion)	
Estazolam (ProSom)	**Zaleplon** (Sonata)	
Eszopiclone (Lunesta)	**Zolpidem** (Ambien)	

COMMENTS: When given orally, alprazolam, midazolam and triazolam undergo extensive first pass metabolism by CYP3A4 in the gut wall and liver. Many other benzodiazepines are also at least partly metabolized by CYP3A4, and may also interact with CYP3A4 inhibitors. Intravenous midazolam is less affected than when it is given orally, but prolonged sedation may occur. The primary risk of these interactions is impairment of motor skills that could result in falls or motor vehicle accidents.

CLASS 3: ASSESS RISK & TAKE ACTION IF NECESSARY
- *Consider Alternative*:
  Benzodiazepines: Consider other benzodiazepines: **temazepam** (Restoril), **oxazepam** (Serax), and **lorazepam** (Ativan) are largely glucuronidated, and are unlikely to be affected by CYP3A4 inhibitors.
  Antidepressants: **Sertraline** (Zoloft), **citalopram** (Celexa), **escitalopram** (Lexapro), **desvenlafaxine** (Pristiq), **venlafaxine** (Effexor), **paroxetine** (Paxil), and **duloxetine** (Cymbalta) appear less likely to inhibit CYP3A4 than fluvoxamine or nefazodone.
- *Monitor*: Monitor for altered benzodiazepine response if the CYP3A4 inhibitor is initiated, discontinued, or changed in dosage. Warn patients about increased sedative effects.

OBJECT DRUGS		PRECIPITANT DRUGS
Anxiolytics/Hypnotics		**Antimicrobials:**
(CYP3A4 Substrates):	**Flurazepam** (Dalmane)	**Ciprofloxacin** (Cipro)
Alprazolam (Xanax)	**Halazepam** (Paxipam)	**Clarithromycin** (Biaxin)
Buspirone (BuSpar)	**Midazolam** (Versed)	**Erythromycin** (E-Mycin)
Clonazepam (Klonopin)	**Prazepam** (Centrex)	**Fluconazole** (Diflucan)
Clorazepate (Tranxene)	**Quazepam** (Doral)	**Itraconazole** (Sporanox)
Diazepam (Valium)	**Triazolam** (Halcion)	**Ketoconazole** (Nizoral)
Estazolam (ProSom)	**Zaleplon** (Sonata)	**Posaconazole** (Noxafil)
Eszopiclone (Lunesta)	**Zolpidem** (Ambien)	**Quinupristin** (Synercid)
		Telithromycin (Ketek)
		Troleandomycin (TAO)
		Voriconazole (Vfend)

COMMENTS: When given orally, alprazolam, midazolam and triazolam undergo extensive first pass metabolism by CYP3A4 in the gut wall and liver, so CYP3A4 inhibitors can dramatically increase plasma concentrations. Many other benzodiazepines are also partly metabolized by CYP3A4, and may also interact with CYP3A4 inhibitors. Intravenous midazolam is less affected than oral midazolam, but prolonged sedation may occur. The primary risk of these interactions is impairment of motor skills that could result in falls or motor vehicle accidents.

CLASS 3: ASSESS RISK & TAKE ACTION IF NECESSARY
- *Consider Alternative*:
  Azole Antifungals: Fluconazole appears to be a less potent inhibitor of CYP3A4; but in larger doses it also inhibits CYP3A4. **Terbinafine** (Lamisil) does not appear to affect CYP3A4.
  Benzodiazepines: Consider other benzodiazepines: **temazepam** (Restoril), **oxazepam** (Serax), and **lorazepam** (Ativan) are largely glucuronidated, and unlikely to be affected by CYP3A4 inhibitors.
  Macrolide Antibiotics: Unlike erythromycin, clarithromycin and troleandomycin, **azithromycin** (Zithromax) and **dirithromycin*** do not appear to inhibit CYP3A4. (*not available in US)
  Telithromycin: The use of **azithromycin** (Zithromax) or a quinolone antibiotic other than ciprofloxacin should be considered.
- *Monitor*: Monitor for altered benzodiazepine response if CYP3A4 inhibitor is initiated, discontinued or changed in dose. Warn patients about increased sedative effects.

OBJECT DRUGS		PRECIPITANT DRUGS
Anxiolytics/Hypnotics		**Calcium Channel Blockers:**
(CYP3A4 substrates):	**Flurazepam** (Dalmane)	**Diltiazem** (Cardizem)
Alprazolam (Xanax)	**Halazepam** (Paxipam)	**Verapamil** (Isoptin)
Buspirone (BuSpar)	**Midazolam** (Versed)	
Clonazepam (Klonopin)	**Prazepam** (Centrex)	
Clorazepate (Tranxene)	**Quazepam** (Doral)	
Diazepam (Valium)	**Triazolam** (Halcion)	
Estazolam (ProSom)	**Zaleplon** (Sonata)	
Eszopiclone (Lunesta)	**Zolpidem** (Ambien)	

COMMENTS: When given orally, alprazolam, midazolam and triazolam undergo extensive first pass metabolism by CYP3A4 in the gut wall and liver. Many other benzodiazepines are also at least partly metabolized by CYP3A4, and may also interact with CYP3A4 inhibitors. Intravenous midazolam is much less affected than when it is given orally, but prolonged sedation may occur. The primary risk of these interactions is impairment of motor skills that could result in falls or motor vehicle accidents.

CLASS 3: ASSESS RISK & TAKE ACTION IF NECESSARY
* *Consider Alternative*:
   Benzodiazepines: Consider other benzodiazepines: **temazepam** (Restoril), **oxazepam** (Serax), and **lorazepam** (Ativan) are largely glucuronidated, and are unlikely to be affected by CYP3A4 inhibitors.
   Calcium Channel Blockers: Calcium channel blockers other than diltiazem and verapamil are unlikely to inhibit the metabolism of benzodiazepines.
* *Monitor*: Monitor for altered benzodiazepine response if the CYP3A4 inhibitor is initiated, discontinued, or changed in dosage. Warn patients about increased sedative effects.

OBJECT DRUGS	PRECIPITANT DRUGS	
Anxiolytics/Hypnotics	**Enzyme Inhibitors:**	
(CYP3A4 substrates):	**(CYP3A4)**	
Alprazolam (Xanax)	**Amiodarone** (Cordarone)	**Nelfinavir** (Viracept)
Buspirone (BuSpar)	**Amprenavir** (Agenerase)	**Ritonavir** (Norvir)
Clonazepam (Klonopin)	**Aprepitant** (Emend)	**Saquinavir** (Invirase)
Clorazepate (Tranxene)	**Atazanavir** (Reyataz)	**Telaprevir** (Incivek)
Diazepam (Valium)	**Boceprevir** (Victrelis)	
Estazolam (ProSom)	**Ceritinib** (Zykadia)	
Eszopiclone (Lunesta)	**Cobicistat** (Stribild)	
Flurazepam (Dalmane)	**Conivaptan** (Vaprisol)	
Halazepam (Paxipam)	**Cyclosporine** (Neoral)	
Midazolam (Versed)	**Darunavir** (Prezista)	
Prazepam (Centrex)	**Delavirdine** (Rescriptor)	
Quazepam (Doral)	**Grapefruit**	
Triazolam (Halcion)	**Indinavir** (Crixivan)	
Zaleplon (Sonata)	**Lomitapide** (Juxtapid)	
Zolpidem (Ambien)	**Mifepristone** (Korlym)	

COMMENTS: When given orally, alprazolam, midazolam and triazolam, undergo extensive first pass metabolism by CYP3A4 in the gut wall and liver. Many other benzodiazepines are also at least partly metabolized by CYP3A4, and may also interact with CYP3A4 inhibitors. Intravenous midazolam is less affected than when it is given orally, but prolonged sedation has been reported. The primary risk of these interactions is impairment of motor skills that could result in falls or motor vehicle accidents. Some of these combinations are listed as contraindicated by the manufacturer (e.g., amprenavir and atazanavir with midazolam or triazolam).

CLASS 3: ASSESS RISK & TAKE ACTION IF NECESSARY
* *Consider Alternative*:
   Benzodiazepines: Consider other benzodiazepines: **temazepam** (Restoril), **oxazepam** (Serax), and **lorazepam** (Ativan) are largely glucuronidated, and are unlikely to be affected by CYP3A4 inhibitors.
   Grapefruit: Orange juice does not appear to inhibit CYP3A4.
* *Monitor*: Monitor for altered benzodiazepine response if the CYP3A4 inhibitor is initiated, discontinued, or changed in dosage. Warn patients about increased sedative effects.

OBJECT DRUGS	PRECIPITANT DRUGS
Aspirin	**NSAIDs:**
	Ibuprofen (Motrin)
	Indomethacin (Indocin)
	Naproxen (Aleve)

COMMENTS: Ibuprofen, naproxen, and possibly indomethacin may interfere with the ability of aspirin to inhibit platelet aggregation, and some evidence suggests that this may also inhibit the cardioprotective effect of aspirin. The effect was seen when ibuprofen was given 2 hours before aspirin, and when ibuprofen was given in multiple daily doses, but not when ibuprofen was given as a single dose 2 hours after aspirin. It is likely that the effect of the timing of doses is similar for naproxen and indomethacin. Current evidence suggests that the antiplatelet effect of aspirin is not affected by diclofenac, sulindac or meloxicam. Little is known about the effect of other NSAIDs on the antiplatelet effect of aspirin, but one should assume that some of them probably do interact. Celecoxib (and probably other COX-2 inhibitors) and acetaminophen do not affect platelet function or the antiplatelet effect of aspirin.

CLASS 3: ASSESS RISK & TAKE ACTION IF NECESSARY
- *Consider Alternative*: Consider using acetaminophen as an alternative if the NSAID is being used as an analgesic. If an NSAID is needed, consider using **diclofenac** (Voltaren), **meloxicam** (Mobic), **sulindac** (Clinoril), or **celecoxib** (Celebrex). Higher doses of aspirin could also be used without loss of antiplatelet effect.
- *Monitor:* If the ibuprofen, naproxen or indomethacin is only taken once daily or less, giving the NSAID 2 hours after the aspirin would probably minimize the interaction.

OBJECT DRUGS	PRECIPITANT DRUGS	
Azole Antifungals:	**Enzyme Inducers:**	
Itraconazole (Sporanox)	**Barbiturates**	**Phenytoin** (Dilantin)
Ketoconazole (Nizoral)	**Bosentan** (Tracleer)	**Primidone** (Mysoline)
Posaconazole (Noxafil)	**Dexamethasone** (Decadron)	**Rifabutin** (Mycobutin)
Voriconazole (Vfend)	**Carbamazepine** (Tegretol)	**Rifampin** (Rifadin)
	Dabrafenib (Tafinlar)	**Rifapentine** (Priftin)
	Efavirenz (Sustiva)	**St. John's wort**
	Lumacaftor (Orkambi)	
	Nevirapine (Viramune)	
	Oxcarbazepine (Trileptal)	

COMMENTS: Rifampin, carbamazepine, phenytoin (and probably other enzyme inducers) markedly reduce serum concentrations of these antifungals. Due to the large magnitude of the interaction it may be difficult to achieve therapeutic concentrations of these antifungal agents. The azole antifungals may also affect some of the enzyme inducers. For example, the azole antifungals may markedly increase carbamazepine or rifabutin concentrations, and voriconazole can increase efavirenz concentrations.

CLASS 3: ASSESS RISK & TAKE ACTION IF NECESSARY
- *Consider Alternative*:
  Antifungal Agent: Fluconazole (Diflucan) appears less likely to interact than other azole antifungals (because of its extensive renal elimination, it is less affected by enzyme inducers), but some reports suggest that enzyme inducers may also reduce fluconazole efficacy. In one study, rifampin markedly increased the clearance of **terbinafine** (Lamisil), so it may also interact.
- *Monitor:* Be alert for loss of antifungal efficacy, and consider increasing the dose of the azole antifungal. Keep in mind that enzyme induction is usually gradual and may take days to weeks for onset and offset, depending on the specific inducer.

OBJECT DRUGS	PRECIPITANT DRUGS	
Azole Antifungals:	**Gastric Antisecretory Agents:**	
Itraconazole (Sporanox)	**Cimetidine** (Tagamet)	**Nizatidine** (Axid)
Ketoconazole (Nizoral)	**Dexlansoprazole** (Kapidex)	**Omeprazole** (Prilosec)
Posaconazole (Noxafil)	**Esomeprazole** (Nexium)	**Pantoprazole** (Protonix)
	Famotidine (Pepcid)	**Rabeprazole** (Aciphex)
	Lansoprazole (Prevacid)	**Ranitidine** (Zantac)

COMMENTS: Itraconazole, ketoconazole, and posaconazole suspension require gastric acidity to be absorbed. Any agent that increases gastric pH can impair their bioavailability.

CLASS 3: ASSESS RISK & TAKE ACTION IF NECESSARY
- *Consider Alternative*: Consider **fluconazole** (Diflucan), **voriconazole** (Vfend), or **terbinafine** (Lamisil) if suitable for the infection.
- *Circumvent/Minimize*: The bioavailability of **itraconazole solution and posaconazole delayed release tablets** are not affected by changes in gastric pH. If an antisecretory agent is necessary, consider using a larger dose of itraconazole or ketoconazole, with monitoring of antifungal serum concentrations if possible. The administration of the antifungal with **Coca-Cola** or **Pepsi** will acidify the stomach and improve the absorption of the antifungal; however a reduction in bioavailability will still occur.
- *Monitor*: Monitor for reduced antifungal effect if itraconazole, ketoconazole, or posaconazole is used with a gastric antisecretory agents.

OBJECT DRUGS	PRECIPITANT DRUGS
Azole Antifungals:	**Gastric Alkalinizers:**
Itraconazole (Sporanox)	**Antacids**
Ketoconazole (Nizoral)	**Didanosine** (Videx)
Posaconazole (Noxafil)	**Sucralfate** (Carafate)

COMMENTS: Itraconazole, ketoconazole, and posaconazole suspension require gastric acidity to be absorbed. Any agent that increases gastric pH can impair their bioavailability. Sucralfate, although not strictly a gastric alkalinizer, has also been noted to reduce the absorption of itraconazole and ketoconazole.

CLASS 3: ASSESS RISK & TAKE ACTION IF NECESSARY
- *Consider Alternative*: Consider **fluconazole** (Diflucan), **voriconazole** (Vfend) or **terbinafine** (Lamisil) if suitable for the infection.
- *Circumvent/Minimize*: The bioavailability of **itraconazole solution and posaconazole delayed release tablets** are not affected by changes in gastric pH. The interaction does not occur with enteric coated bead formulation of didanosine (Videx EC). Administer itraconazole or ketoconazole 2 or more hours prior to antacid, sucralfate, or didanosine. Wait six hours after gastric alkalinizer administration to give itraconazole or ketoconazole.
- *Monitor*: Monitor for reduced antifungal effect if itraconazole, ketoconazole, or posaconazole is used with a gastric alkalinizer or sucralfate.

OBJECT DRUGS	PRECIPITANT DRUGS
Beta-blockers (CYP2D6 Substrates):	**Antidepressants:**
Carvedilol (Coreg)	Bupropion (Wellbutrin)
Metoprolol (Lopressor)	Duloxetine (Cymbalta)
Nebivolol (Bystolic)	Fluoxetine (Prozac)
Propranolol (Inderal)	Paroxetine (Paxil)
Timolol (Blocadren)	

COMMENTS: Antidepressants that are inhibitors of CYP2D6 can increase the concentration of beta-blockers, potentially resulting in bradycardia, hypotension or heart failure. Rapid metabolizers of CYP2D6 (over 90% of the population) will be at the greatest risk.

CLASS 3: ASSESS RISK & TAKE ACTION IF NECESSARY
* *Consider Alternative*:
  Antidepressant: **Sertraline** (Zoloft), **citalopram** (Celexa), **desvenlafaxine** (Pristiq), and **escitalopram** (Lexapro) are weak inhibitors of CYP2D6, while **venlafaxine** (Effexor) and **fluvoxamine** (Luvox) have little or no effect on CYP2D6.
  Beta-blocker: Select a beta-blocker that is not a CYP2D6 substrate such as **atenolol** (Tenormin) or **nadolol** (Corgard).
* *Monitor*: Monitor for altered beta-blocker effect if inhibitor is initiated, discontinued, or changed in dosage.

OBJECT DRUGS	PRECIPITANT DRUGS
Beta-blockers	**Enzyme Inhibitors (CYP2D6):**
(CYP2D6 Substrates):	Abiraterone (Zytiga)
Carvedilol (Coreg)	Amiodarone (Cordarone)
Metoprolol (Lopressor)	Cimetidine (Tagamet)
Nebivolol (Bystolic)	Cinacalcet (Sensipar)
Propranolol (Inderal)	Clobazam (Onfi)
Timolol (Blocadren)	Diphenhydramine (Benadryl)
	Haloperidol (Haldol)
	Mirabegron (Myrbetriq)
	Propafenone (Rythmol)
	Propoxyphene*
	Quinidine (Quinidex)
	Ritonavir (Norvir)
	Terbinafine (Lamisil)
	Thioridazine (Mellaril)

* Propoxyphene (Darvon) was withdrawn from the US market.

COMMENTS: Inhibitors of CYP2D6 can increase the concentration of beta-blockers, potentially resulting in bradycardia, hypotension or heart failure. Rapid metabolizers of CYP2D6 (over 90% of the population) will be at the greatest risk. Note that because terbinafine has an extraordinarily long terminal half-life, the inhibitory effect of terbinafine on CYP2D6 may last for many weeks after terbinafine is discontinued.

CLASS 3: ASSESS RISK & TAKE ACTION IF NECESSARY
* *Consider Alternative*:
  Cimetidine: Other acid suppressors are unlikely to interact. Consider using **famotidine** (Pepcid), **nizatidine** (Axid), **ranitidine** (Zantac), **dexlansoprazole** (Kapidex), **esomeprazole** (Nexium), **omeprazole** (Prilosec), **lansoprazole** (Prevacid), **rabeprazole** (Aciphex), or **pantoprazole** (Protonix).
  Beta-blocker: Select a beta-blocker that is not a CYP2D6 substrate such as **atenolol** (Tenormin) or **nadolol** (Corgard).
* *Monitor*: Monitor for altered beta-blocker effect if inhibitor is initiated, discontinued, or changed in dosage.

OBJECT DRUGS	PRECIPITANT DRUGS	
Calcium Channel Blockers:	**Enzyme Inducers:**	
Amlodipine (Norvasc)	**Barbiturates**	**Phenytoin** (Dilantin)
Bepridil (Vascor)	**Bosentan** (Tracleer)	**Primidone** (Mysoline)
Diltiazem (Cardizem)	**Carbamazepine** (Tegretol)	**Rifabutin** (Mycobutin)
Felodipine (Plendil)	**Dabrafenib** (Tafinlar)	**Rifampin** (Rifadin)
Isradipine (DynaCirc)	**Dexamethasone** (Decadron)	**Rifapentine** (Priftin)
Nicardipine (Cardene)	**Efavirenz** (Sustiva)	**St. John's wort**
Nifedipine (Procardia)	**Lumacaftor** (Orkambi)	
Nimodipine (Nimotop)	**Nevirapine** (Viramune)	
Nisoldipine (Sular)	**Oxcarbazepine** (Trileptal)	
Nitrendipine (Baypress)		
Verapamil (Isoptin)		

COMMENTS: Rifampin markedly reduces the plasma concentrations of verapamil, diltiazem, nifedipine, and nisoldipine; the effect probably occurs with most other combinations of calcium channel blockers (CCBs) and enzyme inducers. The effect is greater with oral than with parenteral administration of the CCB.

CLASS 3: ASSESS RISK & TAKE ACTION IF NECESSARY
- *Consider Alternative*: It may be difficult to achieve therapeutic serum concentrations of oral CCBs in the presence of enzyme inducers. Thus, if at all possible, use an alternative to either the CCB or the enzyme inducer. Avoid barbiturates if a non-barbiturate alternative is suitable (e.g., benzodiazepine). Theoretically, amlodipine would be less affected than other CCBs, since it undergoes less first-pass metabolism.
- *Monitor*: Monitor for altered CCB effect if inducer is initiated, discontinued, or changed in dosage. Keep in mind that enzyme induction is usually gradual and may take days to weeks for onset and offset, depending on the specific inducer.

OBJECT DRUGS		PRECIPITANT DRUGS
Calcium Channel Blockers:		**Antidepressants:**
Amlodipine (Norvasc)	**Nifedipine** (Procardia)	**Fluvoxamine** (Luvox)
Bepridil (Vascor)	**Nimodipine** (Nimotop)	**Nefazodone**
Diltiazem (Cardizem)	**Nisoldipine** (Sular)	
Felodipine (Plendil)	**Nitrendipine** (Baypress)	
Isradipine (DynaCirc)	**Verapamil** (Isoptin)	
Nicardipine (Cardene)		

COMMENTS: CYP3A4 inhibitors may substantially increase calcium channel blocker (CCB) serum concentrations. Not all combinations of CCBs and CYP3A4 inhibitors have been studied; assume they interact until proven otherwise. Note, however, that the magnitude of interaction can vary considerably depending on the CCB involved. For example, felodipine undergoes extensive first pass metabolism by CYP3A4 and is markedly affected by CYP3A4 inhibition, while amlodipine undergoes considerably less first pass metabolism by CYP3A4 and is much less affected by CYP3A4 inhibition. Fluvoxamine appears to be a modest CYP3A4 inhibitor but may produce increased CCB concentrations.

CLASS 3: ASSESS RISK & TAKE ACTION IF NECESSARY
- *Consider Alternative*: Sertraline (Zoloft), citalopram (Celexa), escitalopram (Lexapro), desvenlafaxine (Pristiq), venlafaxine (Effexor), and paroxetine (Paxil) appear less likely to inhibit CYP3A4 than fluvoxamine. Little is known about the effect of other antidepressants on CCBs.
- *Monitor*: If alternatives are not appropriate, consider reducing CCB dose and monitor for altered CCB response if inhibitor is initiated, discontinued, or changed in dosage. Watch for hypotension or other evidence of excessive CCB effect.

OBJECT DRUGS	PRECIPITANT DRUGS
Calcium Channel Blockers:	**Antimicrobials:**
Amlodipine (Norvasc)	**Ciprofloxacin** (Cipro)
Bepridil (Vascor)	**Clarithromycin** (Biaxin)
Diltiazem (Cardizem)	**Erythromycin** (E-Mycin)
Felodipine (Plendil)	**Fluconazole** (Diflucan)
Isradipine (DynaCirc)	**Itraconazole** (Sporanox)
Nicardipine (Cardene)	**Ketoconazole** (Nizoral)
Nifedipine (Procardia)	**Posaconazole** (Noxafil)
Nimodipine (Nimotop)	**Quinupristin** (Synercid)
Nisoldipine (Sular)	**Telithromycin** (Ketek)
Nitrendipine (Baypress)	**Troleandomycin** (TAO)
Verapamil (Isoptin)	**Voriconazole** (Vfend)

COMMENTS: Calcium channel blockers (CCBs) are metabolized by CYP3A4, so CYP3A4 inhibitors may substantially increase their serum concentrations, thus increasing the risk of hypotension and other adverse cardiovascular effects. Not all combinations of CCBs and CYP3A4 inhibitors have been studied; assume they interact until proven otherwise. Note, however, that the magnitude of interaction can vary considerably depending on the CCB involved. For example, felodipine undergoes extensive first pass metabolism by CYP3A4 and is markedly affected by CYP3A4 inhibition, while amlodipine undergoes considerably less first pass metabolism by CYP3A4 and is much less affected by CYP3A4 inhibition. Short-term use of an azole antifungal (1-2 days) is unlikely to result in a clinically important interaction. Erythromycin and clarithromycin may also have intrinsic effects on cardiac conduction that may increase the risk of hypotension.

CLASS 3: ASSESS RISK & TAKE ACTION IF NECESSARY
- *Consider Alternative:*
Azole Antifungals: Fluconazole appears to be a less potent inhibitor of CYP3A4; but in larger doses it also inhibits CYP3A4. **Terbinafine** (Lamisil) does not appear to affect CYP3A4.
Macrolide Antibiotics: Unlike erythromycin, clarithromycin and troleandomycin, **azithromycin** (Zithromax) and **dirithromycin*** do not appear to inhibit CYP3A4. (*not available in US)
Telithromycin: The use of **azithromycin** (Zithromax) or a quinolone antibiotic other than ciprofloxacin should be considered.
- *Monitor:* If alternatives are not appropriate, consider reducing CCB dose and monitor for altered CCB response if inhibitor is initiated, discontinued, or changed in dosage.

OBJECT DRUGS	PRECIPITANT DRUGS	
Calcium Channel Blockers:	**Enzyme Inhibitors:**	
Amlodipine (Norvasc)	**Amiodarone** (Cordarone)	**Diltiazem** (Cardizem)
Bepridil (Vascor)	**Amprenavir** (Agenerase)	**Dronedarone** (Multaq)
Diltiazem (Cardizem)	**Aprepitant** (Emend)	**Grapefruit**
Felodipine (Plendil)	**Atazanavir** (Reyataz)	**Indinavir** (Crixivan)
Isradipine (DynaCirc)	**Boceprevir** (Victrelis)	**Lomitapide** (Juxtapid)
Nicardipine (Cardene)	**Ceritinib** (Zykadia)	**Mifepristone** (Korlym)
Nifedipine (Procardia)	**Cobicistat** (Stribild)	**Nelfinavir** (Viracept)
Nimodipine (Nimotop)	**Conivaptan** (Vaprisol)	**Ritonavir** (Norvir)
Nisoldipine (Sular)	**Cyclosporine** (Neoral)	**Saquinavir** (Invirase)
Nitrendipine (Baypress)	**Darunavir** (Prezista)	**Telaprevir** (Incivek)
Verapamil (Isoptin)	**Delavirdine** (Rescriptor)	**Verapamil** (Isoptin)

COMMENTS: Calcium channel blockers (CCBs) are metabolized by CYP3A4, so CYP3A4 inhibitors may substantially increase their serum concentrations. Not all combinations of CCBs and CYP3A4 inhibitors have been studied; assume they interact until proven otherwise. Note, however, that the magnitude of interaction can vary considerably depending on the CCB involved. For example, felodipine undergoes extensive first pass metabolism by CYP3A4 and is markedly affected by CYP3A4 inhibition, while amlodipine undergoes considerably less first pass metabolism by CYP3A4 and is much less affected by CYP3A4 inhibition. For example, grapefruit juice substantially increases felodipine concentrations, but has minimal effects on amlodipine.

CLASS 3: ASSESS RISK & TAKE ACTION IF NECESSARY
- *Monitor:* If alternatives are not appropriate, consider reducing CCB dose and monitor for altered CCB response if inhibitor is initiated, discontinued, or changed in dosage.

OBJECT DRUGS	PRECIPITANT DRUGS
Carbamazepine (Tegretol)	**Antidepressants:** **Fluoxetine** (Prozac) **Fluvoxamine** (Luvox) **Nefazodone**

COMMENTS: Inhibition of CYP3A4 by fluvoxamine or nefazodone may result in carbamazepine toxicity. With most CYP3A4 inhibitors, carbamazepine toxicity usually occurs within 2-3 days of starting the inhibitor, but the effect of fluoxetine on carbamazepine is less consistent and may be delayed by 1-2 weeks or longer. It may involve enzymes in addition to CYP3A4, perhaps CYP2C19.

CLASS 3: ASSESS RISK & TAKE ACTION IF NECESSARY
- *Consider Alternative*: **Sertraline** (Zoloft), **citalopram** (Celexa), **escitalopram** (Lexapro), **venlafaxine** (Effexor), and **paroxetine** (Paxil) appear less likely to inhibit CYP3A4 than fluvoxamine. Little is known about the effects of other antidepressants on carbamazepine.
- *Monitor*: If alternatives are not appropriate, consider reducing carbamazepine dose. Monitor for altered carbamazepine effect if enzyme inhibitors are started, stopped, or changed in dosage. Symptoms of carbamazepine toxicity include nausea, vomiting, dizziness, drowsiness, headache, diplopia, and confusion.

OBJECT DRUGS	PRECIPITANT DRUGS	
Carbamazepine (Tegretol)	**Antimicrobials:**	
	Ciprofloxacin (Cipro)	**Posaconazole** (Noxafil)
	Clarithromycin (Biaxin)	**Quinupristin** (Synercid)
	Erythromycin (E-Mycin)	**Telithromycin** (Ketek)
	Fluconazole (Diflucan)	**Troleandomycin** (TAO)
	Itraconazole (Sporanox)	**Voriconazole** (Vfend)
	Ketoconazole (Nizoral)	

COMMENTS: Inhibition of CYP3A4 (and possibly other enzymes) by these antimicrobials may result in carbamazepine toxicity, usually within 2-3 days of starting the inhibitor. Adverse outcomes from these interactions are fairly predictable, and most patients who start a CYP3A4 inhibitor while on carbamazepine will develop clinical evidence of carbamazepine toxicity. **Metronidazole** (Flagyl) has also been reported to cause carbamazepine toxicity in isolated cases, but more study is needed.

CLASS 3: ASSESS RISK & TAKE ACTION IF NECESSARY
- *Consider Alternative*:
  Azole Antifungals: Fluconazole appears to be a less potent inhibitor of CYP3A4; but in larger doses it also inhibits CYP3A4. **Terbinafine** (Lamisil) does not appear to affect CYP3A4.
  Macrolide Antibiotics: Unlike erythromycin, clarithromycin and troleandomycin, **azithromycin** (Zithromax) and **dirithromycin*** do not appear to inhibit CYP3A4. (*not available in US)
  Telithromycin: The use of **azithromycin** (Zithromax) or a quinolone antibiotic other than ciprofloxacin should be considered.
- *Monitor*: If alternatives are not appropriate, consider reducing carbamazepine dose. Monitor for altered carbamazepine effect if enzyme inhibitors are started, stopped or changed in dosage. Symptoms of carbamazepine toxicity include nausea, vomiting, dizziness, drowsiness, headache, diplopia, and confusion.

OBJECT DRUGS	PRECIPITANT DRUGS
Carbamazepine (Tegretol)	**Calcium Channel Blockers:** **Diltiazem** (Cardizem) **Verapamil** (Isoptin)

COMMENTS: Inhibition of CYP3A4 by these calcium channel blockers may result in carbamazepine toxicity, usually within 2-3 days of starting the inhibitor. Adverse outcomes from these interactions are fairly predictable, and most patients who start a CYP3A4 inhibitor while on carbamazepine will develop clinical evidence of carbamazepine toxicity. Keep in mind also that enzyme inducers such as carbamazepine can markedly reduce plasma concentrations of most calcium channel blockers.

CLASS 3: ASSESS RISK & TAKE ACTION IF NECESSARY
- *Consider Alternative:* Diltiazem, verapamil, and possibly nicardipine are the only calcium channel blockers (CCBs) known to inhibit CYP3A4; other CCBs are probably less likely to cause carbamazepine toxicity.
- *Monitor:* If alternatives are not appropriate, consider reducing the dose of carbamazepine. Monitor for altered carbamazepine effect if enzyme inhibitors are initiated, discontinued, or changed in dosage. Symptoms of carbamazepine toxicity include nausea, vomiting, dizziness, drowsiness, headache, diplopia, and confusion.

OBJECT DRUGS	PRECIPITANT DRUGS	
Carbamazepine (Tegretol)	**Enzyme Inhibitors:**	
	Amiodarone (Cordarone)	**Delavirdine** (Rescriptor)
	Amprenavir (Agenerase)	**Dronedarone** (Multaq)
	Aprepitant (Emend)	**Grapefruit**
	Atazanavir (Reyataz)	**Indinavir** (Crixivan)
	Boceprevir (Victrelis)	**Isoniazid** (INH)
	Ceritinib (Zykadia)	**Lomitapide** (Juxtapid)
	Cimetidine (Tagamet)	**Mifepristone** (Korlym)
	Cobicistat (Stribild)	**Nelfinavir** (Viracept)
	Conivaptan (Vaprisol)	**Ritonavir** (Norvir)
	Cyclosporine (Neoral)	**Saquinavir** (Invirase)
	Danazol (Danocrine)	**Telaprevir** (Incivek)
	Darunavir (Prezista)	

COMMENTS: Inhibition of CYP3A4 can result in carbamazepine toxicity, usually within 2-3 days of starting the inhibitor; most patients who start a CYP3A4 inhibitor while on carbamazepine will develop clinical evidence of carbamazepine toxicity. The effect of danazol may be delayed by 1-2 weeks. Not all known CYP3A4 inhibitors have been studied with carbamazepine, but assume they interact until proven otherwise.

CLASS 3: ASSESS RISK & TAKE ACTION IF NECESSARY
- *Consider Alternative:*
  Cimetidine: **Famotidine** (Pepcid), **nizatidine** (Axid), and **ranitidine** (Zantac) have minimal effects on drug metabolism.
  Grapefruit: Orange juice does not appear to inhibit CYP3A4.
- *Monitor:* If alternatives are not appropriate, consider reducing the dose of carbamazepine. Monitor for altered carbamazepine effect if enzyme inhibitors are initiated, discontinued, or changed in dosage. Symptoms of carbamazepine toxicity include nausea, vomiting, dizziness, drowsiness, headache, diplopia, and confusion.

OBJECT DRUGS	PRECIPITANT DRUGS	
Central Alpha-adrenergic Agonists:	**Antidepressants:**	
Clonidine (Catapres)	**Amitriptyline** (Elavil)	**Imipramine** (Tofranil)
Guanabenz (Wytensin)	**Amoxapine** (Asendin)	**Mirtazapine** (Remeron)
Guanfacine (Tenex)	**Clomipramine** (Anafranil)	**Nortriptyline** (Aventyl)
	Desipramine (Norpramin)	**Protriptyline** (Vivactil)
	Doxepin (Sinequan)	**Trimipramine** (Surmontil)
	Duloxetine (Cymbalta)	

COMMENTS: Tricyclic antidepressants (TCAs) can markedly reduce the antihypertensive effects of clonidine, guanfacine, and probably guanabenz. The effect is usually gradual but rapid increases in blood pressure have occurred. Also, stopping clonidine-like drugs abruptly in the presence of TCAs may result in an acute hypertensive reaction.

CLASS 2: USE ONLY IF BENEFIT FELT TO OUTWEIGH RISK

- *Use Alternative*:
  Antidepressant: Limited evidence suggests that **trazodone** (Desyrel) may also inhibit the effect of clonidine. Theoretically, serotonin-norepinephrine reuptake inhibitors (SNRI) such as **desvenlafaxine** (Pristiq), **duloxetine** (Cymbalta), **milnacipran** (Savella), and **venlafaxine** (Effexor) would also be expected to inhibit the antihypertensive effects of clonidine-like drugs, so SNRIs may not be suitable alternatives. Little is known regarding the effect of other antidepressants, but use alternative antidepressants only with careful blood pressure monitoring. Antihypertensives: Beta-adrenergic blockers, diuretics, ACEIs, ARBs, and calcium channel blockers appear to be minimally affected by TCAs. Be alert to the potential for **diltiazem** (Cardizem) and **verapamil** (Calan) to inhibit the metabolism of some TCAs. The efficacy of **guanethidine** (Ismelin) and **guanadrel** (Hylorel) is also inhibited by TCAs.
- *Circumvent/Minimize*: In patients receiving central alpha agonists and TCAs, clonidine-like drugs should be tapered instead of stopped abruptly to reduce the likelihood of a hypertensive reaction.
- *Monitor*: In patients on central alpha-receptor agonists, monitor blood pressure carefully if TCAs are initiated, discontinued, or changed in dosage.

OBJECT DRUGS	PRECIPITANT DRUGS
Central Alpha-adrenergic Agonists:	**Yohimbine**
Clonidine (Catapres)	
Guanabenz (Wytensin)	
Guanfacine (Tenex)	

COMMENTS: Yohimbine acts through inhibition of alpha-2 adrenergic receptors, while central alpha-adrenergic agonists stimulate those same receptors. As a result of this pharmacologic antagonism, it is likely that yohimbine will inhibit the antihypertensive effect of clonidine, guanabenz, and guanfacine.

CLASS 2: USE ONLY IF BENEFIT FELT TO OUTWEIGH RISK

- *Use Alternative:* If yohimbine is being used as an "herbal Viagra" in a patient on clonidine, guanabenz, or guanfacine, it would be prudent to use an alternative drug for erectile dysfunction, such as phosphodiesterase inhibitors: **sildenafil** (Viagra), **tadalafil** (Cialis), or **vardenafil** (Levitra). Unlike yohimbine, phosphodiesterase inhibitors may *increase* the antihypertensive effect of clonidine, guanabenz, or guanfacine. Monitor blood pressure.
- *Monitor*: If yohimbine is used with clonidine, guanabenz, or guanfacine, monitor blood pressure for evidence of reduced antihypertensive effect.

OBJECT DRUGS	PRECIPITANT DRUGS	
Cephalosporin Antibiotics:	**Gastric Alkalinizers:**	
Cefditoren (Spectracef)	**Antacids**	**Nizatidine** (Axid)
Cefpodoxime (Vantin)	**Cimetidine** (Tagamet)	**Omeprazole** (Prilosec)
Cefuroxime (Ceftin)	**Dexlansoprazole** (Kapidex)	**Pantoprazole** (Protonix)
	Esomeprazole (Nexium)	**Rabeprazole** (Aciphex)
	Famotidine (Pepcid)	**Ranitidine** (Zantac)
	Lansoprazole (Prevacid)	

COMMENTS: Increasing gastric pH inhibits the absorption of cefditoren, cefpodoxime, and cefuroxime. A loss of efficacy could result in some patients.

CLASS 3: ASSESS RISK & TAKE ACTION IF NECESSARY

Circumvent/Minimize: Administration of the cephalosporin 2 hours before the antacid would minimize the interaction. It may be difficult to separate the doses of an H_2-receptor antagonist or proton pump inhibitor to ensure that no interaction occurs.

- *Consider Alternative*: H_2-receptor antagonists do not affect **cefixime** (Suprax) absorption; theoretically it would also be unaffected by proton pump inhibitors. Other cephalosporins are not known to manifest pH-dependent absorption.
- *Monitor*: Watch for reduced antibiotic efficacy when these cephalosporins are coadministered with gastric alkalinizers.

OBJECT DRUGS	PRECIPITANT DRUGS	
Cholinesterase Inhibitors:	**Antihistamines:**	
Donepezil (Aricept)	**Azatadine** (Optimine)	**Cyproheptadine** (Periactin)
Galantamine (Razadyne)	**Azelastine** (Astelin)	**Dexchlorpheniramine**
Rivastigmine (Exelon)	**Brompheniramine** (Dimetapp)	(Polaramine)
	Chlorpheniramine	**Hydroxyzine** (Atarax)
	(Chlor-Trimeton)	**Promethazine** (Phenergan)
	Clemastine (Tavist)	**Triprolidine** (Actidil)

COMMENTS: The cholinesterase inhibitors used to treat Alzheimer's dementia are cholinergic, while the antihistamines listed above are anticholinergic. Thus, one would expect that these antihistamines would inhibit the efficacy of cholinesterase inhibitors. The clinical evidence suggests that this may occur. Short-term use of the antihistamines may be less likely to cause problems.

CLASS 3: ASSESS RISK & TAKE ACTION IF NECESSARY
• *Consider Alternative*: Consider using an antihistamine with little or no anticholinergic effects, such as **cetirizine** (Zyrtec), **desloratadine** (Clarinex), **ebastine** (Kestine), **fexofenadine** (Allegra), or **loratadine** (Claritin).
• *Monitor*: If the combination is used, monitor for evidence of reduced efficacy of the cholinesterase inhibitor.

OBJECT DRUGS	PRECIPITANT DRUGS	
Cholinesterase Inhibitors:	**Antidepressants, Tricyclic:**	
Donepezil (Aricept)	**Amitriptyline** (Elavil)	**Imipramine** (Tofranil)
Galantamine (Razadyne)	**Amoxapine** (Asendin)	**Nortriptyline** (Aventyl)
Rivastigmine (Exelon)	**Clomipramine** (Anafranil)	**Protriptyline** (Vivactil)
	Desipramine (Norpramin)	**Trimipramine** (Surmontil)
	Doxepin (Sinequan)	

COMMENTS: The cholinesterase inhibitors used to treat Alzheimer's dementia are cholinergic, while tricyclic antidepressants are anticholinergic. Thus, one would expect that these antidepressants would inhibit the efficacy of cholinesterase inhibitors. The clinical evidence suggests that this may occur. Note that some tricyclic antidepressants such as amitriptyline and clomipramine may have stronger anticholinergic effects than others such as desipramine and amoxapine.

CLASS 3: ASSESS RISK & TAKE ACTION IF NECESSARY
• *Consider Alternative*: Consider using an antidepressant with little or no anticholinergic effects such as **bupropion** (Wellbutrin), **mirtazapine** (Remeron), **trazodone** (Desyrel), **selective serotonin reuptake inhibitors** (SSRIs) as a class, and **serotonin-norepinephrine reuptake inhibitors** (SNRIs) as a class.
• *Monitor*: If the combination is used, monitor for evidence of reduced efficacy of the cholinesterase inhibitor.

OBJECT DRUGS	PRECIPITANT DRUGS
Cholinesterase Inhibitors:	**Antiemetic Anticholinergics:**
Donepezil (Aricept)	**Cyclizine** (Marezine)
Galantamine (Razadyne)	**Dimenhydrinate** (Dramamine)
Rivastigmine (Exelon)	**Meclizine** (Antivert)
	Prochlorperazine (Compazine)
	Scopolamine (Transderm Scop)

COMMENTS: The cholinesterase inhibitors used to treat Alzheimer's dementia are cholinergic, while the antiemetic drugs listed above are anticholinergic drugs. Thus, one would expect that these antiemetic drugs would inhibit the efficacy of cholinesterase inhibitors. The clinical evidence suggests that this may occur. Short-term use of the antiemetic may be less likely to cause problems.

CLASS 3: ASSESS RISK & TAKE ACTION IF NECESSARY
• *Consider Alternative:* Consider using an alternative to one of the drugs.
• *Monitor*: If the combination is used, monitor for evidence of reduced efficacy of the cholinesterase inhibitor.

OBJECT DRUGS	PRECIPITANT DRUGS
Cholinesterase Inhibitors:	**Anti-Parkinson Anticholinergics:**
Donepezil (Aricept)	**Benztropine** (Cogentin)
Galantamine (Razadyne)	**Biperiden** (Akineton)
Rivastigmine (Exelon)	**Procyclidine** (Kemadrin)
	Trihexyphenidyl (Artane)

COMMENTS: The cholinesterase inhibitors used to treat Alzheimer's dementia are cholinergic, while the anti-Parkinson drugs listed above are anticholinergic drugs. Thus, one would expect that these anti-Parkinson drugs would inhibit the efficacy of cholinesterase inhibitors. The clinical evidence suggests that this may occur.

CLASS 3: ASSESS RISK & TAKE ACTION IF NECESSARY
- *Consider Alternative:* Consider using an alternative to one of the drugs.
- *Monitor:* If the combination is used, monitor for evidence of reduced efficacy of the cholinesterase inhibitor.

OBJECT DRUGS	PRECIPITANT DRUGS
Cholinesterase Inhibitors:	**Antipsychotics:**
Donepezil (Aricept)	**Chlorpromazine** (Thorazine)
Galantamine (Razadyne)	**Clozapine** (Clozaril)
Rivastigmine (Exelon)	**Olanzapine** (Zyprexa)
	Quetiapine (Seroquel)
	Thioridazine (Mellaril)
	Trifluoperazine (Stelazine)

COMMENTS: The cholinesterase inhibitors used to treat Alzheimer's dementia are cholinergic, while the antipsychotic agents listed above have anticholinergic properties. Thus, one would expect that these antipsychotics would inhibit the efficacy of cholinesterase inhibitors. The clinical evidence suggests that this may occur.

CLASS 3: ASSESS RISK & TAKE ACTION IF NECESSARY
- *Consider Alternative:* Consider using an antipsychotic with little or no anticholinergic effects.
- *Monitor:* If the combination is used, monitor for evidence of reduced efficacy of the cholinesterase inhibitor.

OBJECT DRUGS	PRECIPITANT DRUGS	
Cholinesterase Inhibitors:	**Antispasmodics:**	
Donepezil (Aricept)	**Atropine** (Donnatal)	**Hyoscyamine** (Anaspaz)
Galantamine (Razadyne)	**Dicyclomine** (Bentyl)	**Methscopolamine** (Pamine)
Rivastigmine (Exelon)	**Belladonna** (Bellamine)	**Oxybutynin** (Ditropan)
	Clidinium (Quarzan)	**Propantheline**
	Darifenacin (Enablex)	(Pro-Banthine)
	Fesoterodine (Toviaz)	**Solifenacin** (Vesicare)
	Flavoxate (Urispas)	**Tolterodine** (Detrol)
	Glycopyrrolate (Robinul)	**Trospium** (Sanctura)

COMMENTS: The cholinesterase inhibitors used to treat Alzheimer's dementia are cholinergic, while these antispasmodic agents are anticholinergic. Thus, one would expect that these antispasmodics would inhibit the efficacy of cholinesterase inhibitors. The clinical evidence suggests that this may occur.

CLASS 3: ASSESS RISK & TAKE ACTION IF NECESSARY
- *Consider Alternative:* Consider using an alternative to the anticholinergic antispasmodic or the cholinesterase inhibitor.
- *Monitor:* If the combination is used, monitor for evidence of reduced efficacy of the cholinesterase inhibitor.

OBJECT DRUGS	PRECIPITANT DRUGS	
Cholinesterase Inhibitors:	**Beta-Blockers:**	
Donepezil (Aricept)	Acebutolol (Sectral)	Metoprolol (Lopressor)
Galantamine (Razadyne)	Atenolol (Tenormin)	Nadolol (Corgard)
Rivastigmine (Exelon)	Betaxolol (Kerlone)	Nebivolol (Bystolic)
	Bisoprolol (Zebeta)	Penbutolol (Levatol)
	Carteolol (Ocupress)	Pindolol (Visken)
	Carvedilol (Coreg)	Propranolol (Inderal)
	Esmolol (Brevibloc)	Sotalol (Betapace)
	Labetalol (Trandate)	Timolol (Blocadren)
	Levobunolol (Betagan)	

COMMENTS: Cholinesterase inhibitors increase vagal tone, which tends to slow the heart rate. When they are given with other drugs that slow heart rate such as beta-blockers, excessive bradycardia can result. In some cases the combination of cholinesterase inhibitors and bradycardic drugs has been associated with life-threatening reactions, with severe bradycardia, cardiac arrhythmias, and even cardiac arrest. More study is needed to establish the incidence and magnitude of these interactions, but the potential severity of the reactions dictates that the combinations should be used only with close monitoring.

CLASS 2: USE ONLY IF BENEFIT FELT TO OUTWEIGH RISK
- *Use Alternative:* If appropriate for the patient, consider using an alternative to the cholinesterase inhibitor or the beta blocker.
- *Circumvent/Minimize:* In some cases of excessive bradycardia due to cholinesterase inhibitor drug interactions, a cardiac pacemaker has been inserted and the drugs continued.
- *Monitor:* If the combination is used, monitor the heart rate for excessive slowing, and be alert for other adverse effects such as hypotension and fainting.

OBJECT DRUGS	PRECIPITANT DRUGS
Cholinesterase Inhibitors:	**Bradycardic Drugs:**
Donepezil (Aricept)	Ceritinib (Zykadia)
Galantamine (Razadyne)	Digoxin (Lanoxin)
Rivastigmine (Exelon)	

COMMENTS: Cholinesterase inhibitors increase vagal tone, which tends to slow the heart rate. When they are given with other drugs that slow heart rate such as ceritinib or digoxin, excessive bradycardia can result. In some cases the combination of cholinesterase inhibitors and bradycardic drugs has been associated with life-threatening reactions, with severe bradycardia, cardiac arrhythmias, and even cardiac arrest. More study is needed to establish the importance of these interactions, but the potential severity of the reactions dictates that the combinations should be used only with close monitoring.

CLASS 2: USE ONLY IF BENEFIT FELT TO OUTWEIGH RISK
- *Use Alternative:* If appropriate for the patient, consider using an alternative to the cholinesterase inhibitor or the bradycardic drug.
- *Circumvent/Minimize:* In some cases of excessive bradycardia due to cholinesterase inhibitor drug interactions, a cardiac pacemaker has been inserted and the drugs continued.
- *Monitor:* If the combination is used, monitor the heart rate for excessive slowing, and be alert for other adverse effects such as lightheadedness, dizziness, hypotension and fainting.

OBJECT DRUGS	PRECIPITANT DRUGS
Cholinesterase Inhibitors:	**Muscle Relaxants:**
Donepezil (Aricept)	**Cyclobenzaprine** (Flexeril)
Galantamine (Razadyne)	**Methocarbamol** (Robaxin)
Rivastigmine (Exelon)	**Orphenadrine** (Norflex)

COMMENTS: The cholinesterase inhibitors used to treat Alzheimer's dementia are cholinergic, while the muscle relaxants listed above have anticholinergic properties. Thus, one would expect that these muscle relaxants would inhibit the efficacy of cholinesterase inhibitors. The clinical evidence suggests that this may occur. Short-term use of these muscle relaxants may be less likely to cause problems.

CLASS 3: ASSESS RISK & TAKE ACTION IF NECESSARY
- *Consider Alternative*: Consider using a muscle relaxant with little or no anticholinergic effects.
- *Monitor*: If the combination is used, monitor for evidence of reduced efficacy of the cholinesterase inhibitor.

OBJECT DRUGS	PRECIPITANT DRUGS	
Clopidogrel (Plavix)	**Chloramphenicol**	**Fluvoxamine** (Luvox)
	Cimetidine (Tagamet)	**Isoniazid** (INH)
	Delavirdine (Rescriptor)	**Omeprazole** (Prilosec)
	Efavirenz (Sustiva)	**Ticlopidine** (Ticlid)
	Esomeprazole (Nexium)	**Voriconazole** (Vfend)
	Fluoxetine (Prozac)	

COMMENTS: Inhibitors of CYP2C19 may reduce the metabolism of clopidogrel to its active metabolite. Some reduction in antiplatelet activity and clinical efficacy may occur. Inhibitors of other enzymes that metabolize clopidogrel to its active metabolite (CYP3A4, CYP2C9) may also reduce the efficacy of clopidogrel.

CLASS 3: ASSESS RISK & TAKE ACTION IF NECESSARY
- *Consider Alternative:* Other PPIs may be less likely to interact with clopidogrel than omeprazole or esomeprazole.
- *Monitor*: Monitor for reduced antiplatelet activity in patients taking clopidogrel and drugs that inhibit its conversion to the active metabolite.

OBJECT DRUGS	PRECIPITANT DRUGS
Codeine Derivatives:	**Antidepressants:**
Codeine	**Bupropion** (Wellbutrin)
Dihydrocodeine (Synalgos-DC)	**Duloxetine** (Cymbalta)
Hydrocodone (Vicodin, Lortab)	**Fluoxetine** (Prozac)
Oxycodone (Percodan, Percocet)	**Paroxetine** (Paxil)

COMMENTS: Antidepressants that inhibit CYP2D6 prevent the conversion of codeine to its active metabolite, morphine; inhibition of analgesic effect may result. Preliminary evidence suggests that the analgesic effect of hydrocodone, oxycodone, and dihydrocodeine is also inhibited with reduced CYP2D6 activity. The analgesic effect of **tramadol** (Ultram) appears to be only partially dependent on CYP2D6, and thus it may have some analgesic activity in the presence of CYP2D6 inhibitors.

CLASS 3: ASSESS RISK & TAKE ACTION IF NECESSARY
- *Consider Alternative*:
  Analgesic: Consider using an analgesic that does not require conversion to an active metabolite, e.g., **morphine**, **methadone** (Dolophine), **fentanyl** (Duragesic), **hydromorphone** (Dilaudid), **butorphanol** (Stadol), or **oxymorphone** (Numorphan).
  Antidepressant: **Citalopram** (Celexa), **escitalopram** (Lexapro), and **sertraline** (Zoloft) are weak inhibitors of CYP2D6, **desvenlafaxine** (Pristiq), **venlafaxine** (Effexor) and **fluvoxamine** (Luvox) have little or no effect on CYP2D6
- *Monitor*: Monitor for loss of analgesic efficacy.

40

OBJECT DRUGS	PRECIPITANT DRUGS	
Codeine Derivatives:	**Enzyme Inhibitors:**	
Codeine	**Abiraterone** (Zytiga)	**Mirabegron** (Myrbetriq)
Dihydrocodeine (Synalgos-DC)	**Amiodarone** (Cordarone)	**Propafenone** (Rythmol)
Hydrocodone (Vicodin, Lortab)	**Cimetidine** (Tagamet)	**Propoxyphene***
Oxycodone (Percodan)	**Cinacalcet** (Sensipar)	**Quinidine** (Quinidex)
	Clobazam (Onfi)	**Ritonavir** (Norvir)
	Diphenhydramine (Benadryl)	**Terbinafine** (Lamisil)
	Haloperidol (Haldol)	**Thioridazine** (Mellaril)

* Propoxyphene (Darvon) was withdrawn from the US market.

COMMENTS: Inhibitors of CYP2D6 prevent the conversion of codeine to its active metabolite, morphine; inhibition of analgesic effect may result. Preliminary evidence suggests that the analgesic effect of hydrocodone, oxycodone, and dihydrocodeine is also reduced in the absence of CYP2D6 activity. The analgesic effect of **tramadol** (Ultram) appears to be only partially dependent on CYP2D6, and thus it may have some analgesic activity in the presence of CYP2D6 inhibitors. Note that because terbinafine has an extraordinarily long terminal half-life, the inhibitory effect of terbinafine on CYP2D6 may last for many weeks after terbinafine is discontinued.

CLASS 3: ASSESS RISK & TAKE ACTION IF NECESSARY
* *Consider Alternative*:
  Analgesic: Consider using an analgesic that does not require conversion to an active metabolite, e.g., **morphine**, **methadone** (Dolophine), **fentanyl** (Duragesic), **hydromorphone** (Dilaudid), **butorphanol** (Stadol), or **oxymorphone** (Numorphan).
  Cimetidine: Other H_2-receptor antagonists such as **famotidine** (Pepcid), **nizatidine** (Axid), or **ranitidine** (Zantac) may be substituted for cimetidine.
* *Monitor*: Monitor for loss of analgesic efficacy.

OBJECT DRUGS	PRECIPITANT DRUGS	
Colchicine (Colcrys)	**Antimicrobials:**	
	Ciprofloxacin (Cipro)	**Posaconazole** (Noxafil)
	Clarithromycin (Biaxin)	**Quinupristin** (Synercid)
	Erythromycin (E-Mycin)	**Telithromycin** (Ketek)
	Fluconazole (Diflucan)	**Troleandomycin** (TAO)
	Itraconazole (Sporanox)	**Voriconazole** (Vfend)
	Ketoconazole (Nizoral)	

COMMENTS: Colchicine is a substrate for CYP3A4 and P-glycoprotein (P-gp) and concurrent use of CYP3A4 and P-gp inhibitors has resulted in severe colchicine toxicity, including gastrointestinal toxicity, rhabdomyolysis, pancytopenia, and multi-organ failure. Colchicine toxicity is difficult to treat, and fatalities have been reported. Most of the antimicrobials above inhibit both CYP3A4 and P-gp, and it has not been established that drugs inhibiting only one or the other would increase colchicine plasma levels. For example, voriconazole inhibits CYP3A4 but may not have much effect on P-gp, so it is possible that it is less likely to interact with colchicine than drugs that inhibit both.

CLASS 2: USE ONLY IF BENEFIT FELT TO OUTWEIGH RISK
* *Use Alternative*: Colchicine toxicity can be fatal, and few situations warrant the use of a CYP3A4/PGP inhibitor with colchicine. Select an alternative that is not known to inhibit PGP or CYP3A4, especially if the patient has renal impairment.
  Azole Antifungals: **Terbinafine** (Lamisil) does not appear to affect CYP3A4, and is not known to inhibit P-glycoprotein, but monitor for colchicine toxicity if it is used.
  Macrolide Antibiotics: Unlike erythromycin, clarithromycin and troleandomycin, **azithromycin** (Zithromax) does not appear to inhibit CYP3A4. But it may weakly inhibit P-glycoprotein, so monitor for colchicine toxicity if it is used.
  Telithromycin: The use of **azithromycin** (Zithromax) or a quinolone antibiotic other than ciprofloxacin should be considered.
* *Monitor*: If the combination must be used, monitor carefully for toxicity from colchicine including diarrhea, fever, abdominal pain, muscle pain or weakness, and paresthesias. Discontinue both drugs immediately if toxicity is suspected.

OBJECT DRUGS	PRECIPITANT DRUGS	
Colchicine (Colcrys)	**Inhibitors of CYP3A4 and P-glycoprotein:**	
	Amiodarone (Cordarone)	**Lapatinib** (Tykerb)
	Aprepitant (Emend)	**Lomitapide** (Juxtapid)
	Atazanavir (Reyataz)	**Mifepristone** (Korlym)
	Boceprevir (Victrelis)	**Nefazodone**
	Ceritinib (Zykadia)	**Nelfinavir** (Viracept)
	Cobicistat (Stribild)	**Nicardipine** (Cardene)
	Conivaptan (Vaprisol)	**Paritaprevir** (Technivie)
	Cyclosporine (Neoral)	**Propafenone** (Rythmol)
	Daclatasvir (Daklinza)	**Quinidine** (Quinidex)
	Delavirdine (Rescriptor)	**Ritonavir** (Norvir)
	Diltiazem (Cardizem)	**Saquinavir** (Invirase)
	Dronedarone (Multaq)	**Tacrolimus** (Prograf)
	Grapefruit	**Tamoxifen** (Nolvadex)
	Indinavir (Crixivan)	**Telaprevir** (Incivek)
		Verapamil (Isoptin)

COMMENTS: Colchicine is a substrate for CYP3A4 and P-glycoprotein (P-gp) and concurrent use of CYP3A4 and P-gp inhibitors has resulted in severe colchicine toxicity, including gastrointestinal toxicity, rhabdomyolysis, pancytopenia, and multi-organ failure. Colchicine toxicity is difficult to treat, and fatalities have been reported, especially if the patient has renal impairment. Most of the inhibitors listed above inhibit both CYP3A4 and P-gp, and it has not been established that drugs inhibiting only one or the other would increase colchicine plasma levels. For example, propafenone inhibits P-gp but may not have much effect on CYP3A4, so it is possible that it is less likely to interact with colchicine than drugs that inhibit both. Although grapefruit inhibits both CYP3A4 and P-gp, and colchicine toxicity has been reported with large amounts of grapefruit juice, one study failed to find an effect of grapefruit juice on colchicine.

CLASS 2: USE ONLY IF BENEFIT FELT TO OUTWEIGH RISK
- *Use Alternative*: Given the possibility of fatal colchicine toxicity, few situations would warrant the use of a PGP or CYP3A4 inhibitor with colchicine. Select an alternative that is not known to inhibit PGP or CYP3A4.
  Calcium Channel Blockers: Calcium channel blockers other than diltiazem, nicardipine, and verapamil appear less likely to inhibit CYP3A4, and may be less likely to inhibit P-glycoprotein. But monitor for colchicine toxicity if any calcium channel blocker is used concurrently.
  Grapefruit: Orange juice does not appear to inhibit CYP3A4.
- *Monitor*: If the combination must be used, monitor carefully for toxicity from colchicine including diarrhea, fever, abdominal pain, muscle pain or weakness, and paresthesias. Discontinue both drugs immediately if toxicity is suspected.

OBJECT DRUGS	PRECIPITANT DRUGS	
Contraceptives, Oral	**Enzyme Inducers:**	
	Armodafinil (Nuvigil)	**Nelfinavir** (Viracept)*
	Barbiturates	**Nevirapine** (Viramune)
	Bexarotene (Targretin)	**Oxcarbazepine** (Trileptal)
	Bosentan (Tracleer)	**Perampanel** (Fycompa)
	Carbamazepine (Tegretol)	**Phenytoin** (Dilantin)
	Dabrafenib (Tafinlar)	**Primidone** (Mysoline)
	Deferasirox (Exjade)	**Rifabutin** (Mycobutin)
	Dexamethasone (Decadron)	**Rifampin** (Rifadin)
	Efavirenz (Sustiva)	**Rifapentine** (Priftin)
	Lumacaftor (Orkambi)	**Ritonavir** (Norvir)
	Felbamate (Felbatol)	**Rufinamide** (Banzel)
	Griseofulvin (Fulvicin)	**St. John's wort**
	Modafinil (Provigil)	**Topiramate** (Topamax)

* Nelfinavir is an *inhibitor* of CYP3A4, but can substantially reduce concentrations of ethinyl estradiol, possibly by induction of glucuronidation and/or CYP2C9.

COMMENTS: Enzyme inducers increase the risk of ovulation and unintended pregnancy in women receiving oral contraceptives. Felbamate may reduce levels of gestodene but not ethinyl estradiol. Bexarotene and bosentan are both known teratogens. At least one case of unintended pregnancy has been reported in a patient using an implantable hormonal contraceptive (Implanon) who took carbamazepine concurrently. The effect of modafinil appears modest, but could increase the risk of contraceptive failure in some people. Keep in mind that enzyme induction is usually gradual and may take days to weeks for onset and offset, depending on the specific inducer. Rufinamide is a mild inducer of CYP3A4, but may reduce the concentrations of ethinyl estradiol and norethindrone. Perampanel (12 mg/day) reduced levonorgestrel AUC by 40%, so consider the possibility that perampanel can reduce the efficacy of hormonal contraceptives.

CLASS 2: USE ONLY IF BENEFIT FELT TO OUTWEIGH RISK

- *Use Alternative:* Use an alternative to the enzyme inducer if possible. If the enzyme inducer is necessary consider adding alternative contraception.
  Anticonvulsants: Agents that may be less likely to interact with oral contraceptives include **gabapentin** (Neurontin), **levetiracetam** (Keppra), **pregabalin** (Lyrica), **tiagabine** (Gabitril), and **valproate** (Depakote). Oral contraceptives may substantially reduce plasma concentrations of **lamotrigine** (Lamictal).
  Oral Contraceptives: Some evidence suggests that enzyme inducers may have less effect on other forms of contraception such as depo-medroxyprogesterone acetate or levonorgestrel-releasing intrauterine systems. Consult current prescribing information.
- *Circumvent/Minimize:* If enzyme inducers are used with oral contraceptives, contraceptive dose may need to be increased. Nonetheless, increases in oral contraceptive dose do not guarantee contraceptive efficacy. When using oral contraceptives with enzyme inducers, patients should use an alternative method of birth control for one cycle after discontinuation of the inducer.
- *Monitor:* Menstrual irregularities (spotting, breakthrough bleeding) may be a sign of inadequate contraceptive hormone levels, but absence of menstrual problems does not guarantee adequate contraception.

OBJECT DRUGS	PRECIPITANT DRUGS	
Contraceptives, Oral	**Antibiotics, Oral:**	
	Amoxicillin (Amoxil)	**Tetracyclines**
	Ampicillin	**Other Oral Antibiotics**

COMMENTS: (See Contraceptives, Oral + Enzyme Inducers for rifabutin, rifapentine, and rifampin). Menstrual irregularities and (rarely) unintended pregnancies have occurred during or after oral antibiotic therapy in women on oral contraceptives. The antibiotics most often implicated are ampicillin (and related penicillins) and tetracyclines, but isolated cases have occurred with many antibiotics. This interaction is controversial; evidence supporting the interaction is largely anecdotal, but most negative studies are also flawed. Although a causal relationship has not been established, assume that the interaction occurs until proven otherwise. Theoretically antibiotics that inhibit CYP3A4 (e.g., erythromycin or clarithromycin) would inhibit estrogen and progestin metabolism, thus *decreasing* the likelihood of reduced contraceptive efficacy.

CLASS 3: ASSESS RISK & TAKE ACTION IF NECESSARY

- *Circumvent/Minimize:* Patients receiving oral contraceptives should be warned about the possibility of reduced efficacy if oral antibiotics are taken. It would be prudent to add other contraception during antibiotic therapy and for at least one cycle after the antibiotic is discontinued.
- *Monitor:* Menstrual irregularities (spotting, breakthrough bleeding) may be a sign of inadequate contraceptive hormone levels, but absence of menstrual problems does not guarantee adequate contraception.

OBJECT DRUGS	PRECIPITANT DRUGS
Corticosteroids:	**Antimicrobials:**
Budesonide (Entocort)	**Ciprofloxacin** (Cipro)
Cortisone (Cortone)	**Clarithromycin** (Biaxin)
Dexamethasone (Decadron)	**Erythromycin** (E-Mycin)
Fluticasone (Flovent)	**Fluconazole** (Diflucan)
Methylprednisolone (Medrol)	**Itraconazole** (Sporanox)
Mometasone (Asmanex)	**Ketoconazole** (Nizoral)
Prednisolone (Prelone)	**Posaconazole** (Noxafil)
Prednisone (Orasone)	**Telithromycin** (Ketek)
Triamcinolone (Aristocort)	**Troleandomycin** (TAO)
	Voriconazole (Vfend)

COMMENTS: Inhibition of CYP3A4 by these antimicrobials may result in substantial increases in the plasma concentrations of these corticosteroids. This can lead to Cushing's syndrome and adrenal suppression. Although inhaled budesonide or fluticasone are not intended to act systemically, numerous cases have been reported of Cushing's syndrome and adrenal insufficiency due to concurrent use of potent CYP3A4 inhibitors such as itraconazole and ritonavir.

CLASS 3: ASSESS RISK & TAKE ACTION IF NECESSARY
- *Consider Alternative*:
  Corticosteroids: Clinical evidence suggests that prednisone and prednisolone are less affected by CYP3A4 inhibitors, but one should still be alert for evidence of corticosteroid toxicity. Theoretically, beclomethasone is unlikely to be affected by CYP3A4 inhibitors.
  Azole Antifungals: Itraconazole and ketoconazole are potent inhibitors of CYP3A4; fluconazole appears weaker, but in larger doses it also inhibits CYP3A4. **Terbinafine** (Lamisil) does not appear to affect CYP3A4, and would not be expected to interact with corticosteroids.
  Macrolide Antibiotics: Unlike erythromycin, clarithromycin and troleandomycin, **azithromycin** (Zithromax) and **dirithromycin*** do not appear to inhibit CYP3A4. (*not available in US)
  Telithromycin: The use of **azithromycin** (Zithromax) or a quinolone antibiotic other than ciprofloxacin should be considered.
- *Monitor*: If CYP3A4 inhibitors are used with dexamethasone or methylprednisolone, monitor for evidence of corticosteroid toxicity such as hypertension, edema, diabetes, poor wound healing, mood swings, muscle weakness, ocular toxicity, and Cushing's syndrome (moon face, central obesity, bruising, hirsutism, acne).

OBJECT DRUGS		PRECIPITANT DRUGS
Corticosteroids:		**Antidepressants:**
Budesonide (Entocort)	**Fluticasone** (Flovent)	**Fluvoxamine** (Luvox)
Cortisone (Cortone)	**Methylprednisolone** (Medrol)	**Nefazodone**
Mometasone (Asmanex)	**Prednisolone** (Prelone)	
Dexamethasone	**Prednisone** (Orasone)	
(Decadron)	**Triamcinolone** (Aristocort)	

COMMENTS: Inhibition of CYP3A4 by these antidepressants may result in substantial increases in the plasma concentrations of these corticosteroids, even when the corticosteroids are given nasally or by inhalation. This can lead to Cushing's syndrome and adrenal suppression. Although inhaled budesonide or fluticasone are not intended to act systemically, numerous cases have been reported of Cushing's syndrome and adrenal insufficiency due to concurrent use of potent CYP3A4.

CLASS 3: ASSESS RISK & TAKE ACTION IF NECESSARY
- *Consider Alternative*:
  Corticosteroids: Clinical evidence suggests that prednisone and prednisolone are less affected by CYP3A4 inhibitors, but one should still be alert for evidence of corticosteroid toxicity. Theoretically, beclomethasone is unlikely to be affected by CYP3A4 inhibitors.
  Antidepressants: **Sertraline** (Zoloft), **citalopram** (Celexa), **escitalopram** (Lexapro), **venlafaxine** (Effexor), and **paroxetine** (Paxil) appear less likely to inhibit CYP3A4 than fluvoxamine. **Fluoxetine** (Prozac) appears to be a weak inhibitor of CYP3A4, but little is known about the effect of other antidepressants on corticosteroids.
- *Monitor*: If CYP3A4 inhibitors are used with these corticosteroids, monitor for evidence of corticosteroid toxicity such as hypertension, edema, diabetes, poor wound healing, mood swings, muscle weakness, ocular toxicity, and Cushing's syndrome (moon face, central obesity, bruising, hirsutism, acne).

44

OBJECT DRUGS	PRECIPITANT DRUGS	
Corticosteroids:	**Enzyme Inhibitors:**	
Budesonide (Entocort)	**Amiodarone** (Cordarone)	**Diltiazem** (Cardizem)
Cortisone (Cortone)	**Amprenavir** (Agenerase)	**Dronedarone** (Multaq)
Dexamethasone (Decadron)	**Aprepitant** (Emend)	**Grapefruit**
Fluticasone (Flovent)	**Atazanavir** (Reyataz)	**Indinavir** (Crixivan)
Methylprednisolone (Medrol)	**Boceprevir** (Victrelis)	**Lomitapide** (Juxtapid)
Mometasone (Asmanex)	**Ceritinib** (Zykadia)	**Mifepristone** (Korlym)
Prednisolone (Prelone)	**Cobicistat** (Stribild)	**Nelfinavir** (Viracept)
Prednisone (Orasone)	**Conivaptan** (Vaprisol)	**Ritonavir** (Norvir)
Triamcinolone (Aristocort)	**Cyclosporine** (Neoral)	**Saquinavir** (Invirase)
	Darunavir (Prezista)	**Telaprevir** (Incivek)
	Delavirdine (Rescriptor)	**Verapamil** (Isoptin)

COMMENTS: Inhibition of CYP3A4 may result in substantial increases in the plasma concentrations of these corticosteroids, even when the corticosteroids are given nasally or by inhalation. This can lead to Cushing's syndrome and adrenal suppression. For example, ritonavir was found to dramatically increase plasma fluticasone concentrations, accompanied by marked suppression of endogenous cortisol production. Although inhaled budesonide or fluticasone are not intended to act systemically, numerous cases have appeared of Cushing's syndrome and adrenal insufficiency due to concurrent use of a potent CYP3A4 inhibitor.

CLASS 3: ASSESS RISK & TAKE ACTION IF NECESSARY
• *Consider Alternative*:
Corticosteroids: Clinical evidence suggests that prednisone and prednisolone are less affected by CYP3A4 inhibitors, but one should still be alert for evidence of corticosteroid toxicity. Theoretically, beclomethasone is unlikely to be affected by CYP3A4 inhibitors.
Calcium channel blockers: Calcium channel blockers other than diltiazem and verapamil are unlikely to inhibit CYP3A4.
Grapefruit: Orange juice does not appear to inhibit CYP3A4.
• *Monitor*: If CYP3A4 inhibitors are used with these corticosteroids, monitor for evidence of corticosteroid toxicity such as hypertension, edema, diabetes, poor wound healing, mood swings, muscle weakness, myopathy, ocular toxicity, and Cushing's syndrome (moon face, central obesity, bruising, hirsutism, acne).

OBJECT DRUGS	PRECIPITANT DRUGS	
Corticosteroids:	**Enzyme Inducers:**	
Betamethasone (Celestone)	**Barbiturates**	**Phenytoin** (Dilantin)
Cortisone (Cortone)	**Bosentan** (Tracleer)	**Primidone** (Mysoline)
Dexamethasone (Decadron)	**Carbamazepine** (Tegretol)	**Rifabutin** (Mycobutin)
Hydrocortisone (Cortef)	**Dabrafenib** (Tafinlar)	**Rifampin** (Rifadin)
Methylprednisolone (Medrol)	**Efavirenz** (Sustiva)	**Rifapentine** (Priftin)
Prednisolone (Prelone)	**Lumacaftor** (Orkambi)	**St. John's wort**
Prednisone (Orasone)	**Nevirapine** (Viramune)	**Topiramate** (Topamax)
Triamcinolone (Aristocort)	**Oxcarbazepine** (Trileptal)	

COMMENTS: Enzyme inducers can enhance the metabolism and reduce the therapeutic response to systemic corticosteroids. Increased corticosteroid dosage may be necessary. No adverse interaction would be expected if the corticosteroid is given topically or for other local effect, since reduced systemic exposure to the corticosteroid might actually reduce systemic adverse effects.

CLASS 3: ASSESS RISK & TAKE ACTION IF NECESSARY
• *Monitor*: Monitor the patient for reduced corticosteroid response if enzyme inducers are given concurrently. Substantial alterations in corticosteroid dosage may be necessary if enzyme inducers are initiated, discontinued, or changed in dosage. Keep in mind that enzyme induction is usually gradual and may take days to weeks for onset and offset.

OBJECT DRUGS	PRECIPITANT DRUGS
Corticosteroids:	**Quinolone Antibiotics:**
Betamethasone (Celestone)	**Ciprofloxacin** (Cipro)
Cortisone (Cortone)	**Gemifloxacin** (Factive)
Dexamethasone (Decadron)	**Levofloxacin** (Levaquin)
Hydrocortisone (Cortef)	**Norfloxacin** (Noroxin)
Methylprednisolone (Medrol)	**Ofloxacin** (Floxin
Prednisolone (Prelone)	
Prednisone (Orasone)	
Triamcinolone (Aristocort)	

COMMENTS: Both case reports and case-controlled studies have identified an increased risk of tendon rupture during the coadministration of systemic steroids and quinolone antibiotics. Both classes of drugs have a toxic effect on tenocytes, but via different mechanisms. In addition to the pharmacodynamic interaction between corticosteroids and quinolone antibiotics, quinolones that inhibit the metabolism of corticosteroids (eg, ciprofloxacin) may exhibit a dual interaction mechanism.

CLASS 3: ASSESS RISK & TAKE ACTION IF NECESSARY
- *Monitor:* Patients should avoid excessive tendon stress during the coadministration of steroids and quinolones. Monitor the patient for signs of tendon injury. The interaction appears to be more common in patients over 60 years of age and those with renal insufficiency.

OBJECT DRUGS	PRECIPITANT DRUGS	
Desmopressin (DDAVP)	**NSAIDs:**	
	Diclofenac (Voltaren)	**Meclofenamate**
	Diflunisal (Dolobid)	**Mefenamic acid**
	Etodolac (Lodine)	**Meloxicam** (Mobic)
	Fenoprofen (Nalfon)	**Nabumetone** (Relafen)
	Flurbiprofen (Ansaid)	**Naproxen** (Aleve)
	Ibuprofen (Motrin)	**Oxaprozin** (Daypro)
	Indomethacin (Indocin)	**Piroxicam** (Feldene)
	Ketoprofen (Orudis)	**Sulindac** (Clinoril)
	Ketorolac (Toradol)	**Tolmetin** (Tolectin)

COMMENTS: NSAIDs can potentiate the effects of desmopressin, and severe hyponatremia with coma and seizures has been reported when NSAIDs were added to desmopressin therapy in patients with central diabetes insipidus or von Willebrand's disease. Desmopressin is also used for nocturia in the elderly, and it is not unusual for such patients to take NSAIDs concurrently. It is not known how often combined use of desmopressin and NSAIDs causes hyponatremia, but it may occur primarily in predisposed patients. Many diseases can predispose to hyponatremia, as can a number of drugs (eg, ACE inhibitors, antineoplastics, antipsychotics, SSRIs, diuretics, etc.)

CLASS 2: USE ONLY IF BENEFIT FELT TO OUTWEIGH RISK
- *Use Alternative:*
  NSAIDs: In patients taking desmopressin, it would be prudent to use alternative to NSAIDs when possible. Consider using **acetaminophen** if the NSAID is being used as an analgesic or antipyretic. It is not known if COX-2 inhibitors such **celecoxib** would be less likely than regular NSAIDs to interact with desmopressin, but there have been isolated cases of hyponatremia with desmopressin combined with celecoxib or other COX-2 inhibitors.
- *Monitor:* If NSAIDs are used with desmopressin, monitor carefully for evidence of hyponatremia. Early signs are relatively nonspecific, including weakness, dizziness, headache, confusion, disorientation, nausea, vomiting, and muscle cramps. If hyponatremia is severe, it can lead to seizures, coma and death. In predisposed patients such as elderly women it may be prudent to measure baseline serum sodium and again after the second drug is started. Symptomatic hyponatremia can occur within a day or two of adding an NSAID to desmopressin therapy.

OBJECT DRUGS	PRECIPITANT DRUGS
Digoxin (Lanoxin)	**Calcium Channel Blockers:** **Bepridil** (Vascor) **Diltiazem** (Cardizem) **Verapamil** (Isoptin)

COMMENTS: These calcium channel blockers inhibit P-glycoprotein and may reduce the renal and nonrenal elimination of digoxin. Digoxin plasma concentrations may increase substantially in some patients. Additive inhibition of A-V conduction may also occur. Nonetheless, with proper monitoring, digoxin is often used with these agents with good results.

CLASS 3: ASSESS RISK & TAKE ACTION IF NECESSARY
- *Consider Alternative:* Dihydropyridine calcium channel blockers such as **amlodipine** (Norvasc), **felodipine** (Plendil), or **nifedipine** (Procardia) do not appear to affect digoxin concentrations.
- *Monitor:* Monitor for altered digoxin effect if one of these calcium channel blockers is initiated, discontinued or changed in dosage; adjustments of digoxin dosage may be needed. Up to 10 days may be required for digoxin to achieve a new steady-state. If digoxin is initiated in the presence of therapy with one of these agents, consider conservative doses of digoxin.

OBJECT DRUGS	PRECIPITANT DRUGS	
Digoxin (Lanoxin)	**P-glycoprotein Inhibitors:**	
	Amiodarone (Cordarone)	**Lomitapide** (Juxtapid)
	Azithromycin (Zithromax)	**Nelfinavir** (Viracept)
	Canagliflozin (Invokana)	**Paritaprevir** (Technivie)
	Clarithromycin (Biaxin)	**Posaconazole** (Noxafil)
	Conivaptan (Vaprisol)	**Propafenone** (Rythmol)
	Cyclosporine (Neoral)	**Quinidine** (Quinidex)
	Daclatasvir (Daklinza)	**Ranolazine** (Ranexa)
	Dronedarone (Multaq)	**Ritonavir** (Norvir)
	Erythromycin (E-Mycin)	**Saquinavir** (Invirase)
	Ezogabine (Potiga)	**Sunitinib** (Sutent)
	Hydroxychloroquine	**Tacrolimus** (Prograf)
	Indinavir (Crixivan)	**Tamoxifen** (Nolvadex)
	Itraconazole (Sporanox)	**Telaprevir** (Incivek)
	Ketoconazole (Nizoral)	**Telithromycin** (Ketek)
	Lapatinib (Tykerb)	**Ticagrelor** (Brilinta)

COMMENTS: Inhibitors of P-glycoprotein reduce the renal and nonrenal elimination of digoxin. Digoxin plasma concentrations may increase two- to four-fold but larger increases may occur especially with potent P-glycoprotein inhibitors such as quinidine or amiodarone. Clarithromycin appears to cause greater increases in digoxin plasma concentrations than erythromycin or azithromycin. The mechanism for the substantial increase in digoxin concentrations following concurrent use of hydroxychloroquine is not established. **Carvedilol** (Coreg) may produce small increases in digoxin plasma concentrations, although larger increases have been reported in children. A metabolite of ezogabine inhibits P-glycoprotein and may increase plasma digoxin, but clinical reports are lacking.

CLASS 3: ASSESS RISK & TAKE ACTION IF NECESSARY
- *Consider Alternative:*
  Macrolide Antibiotics: It is not known if dirithromycin* would interact with digoxin. (*not available in US)
- *Monitor:* Monitor for altered digoxin effect if one of these P-glycoprotein inhibitors is initiated, discontinued or changed in dosage; adjustments of digoxin dosage may be needed. Up to 10 days may be required for digoxin to achieve a new steady-state. If digoxin is initiated in the presence of therapy with one of these agents, consider conservative doses of digoxin.

OBJECT DRUGS	PRECIPITANT DRUGS
Digoxin (Lanoxin)	**P-glycoprotein Inducers:** **Carbamazepine** (Tegretol) **Dexamethasone** (Decadron) **Rifampin** (Rimactane) **St. John's wort** **Tipranavir** (Aptivus)

COMMENTS: Rifampin and St. John's wort have been shown to substantially reduce the plasma concentration of digoxin; although data are limited, other P-glycoprotein inducers may have a similar effect on digoxin concentrations. Although some evidence suggests that carbamazepine induces P-gp, one study found no effect of carbamazepine on digoxin serum concentrations. Several days to weeks may be required to see the full effect a P-glycoprotein inducer on digoxin.

CLASS 3: ASSESS RISK & TAKE ACTION IF NECESSARY
Monitor: Monitor for altered digoxin effect if a P-glycoprotein inducer is initiated, discontinued or changed in dosage; adjustments of digoxin dosage may be needed.

OBJECT DRUGS		PRECIPITANT DRUGS
Diuretics:		**Binding Resins:**
Bumetanide (Bumex)	**Thiazides**	**Cholestyramine** (Questran)
Furosemide (Lasix)	**Torsemide** (Demadex)	**Colestipol** (Colestid)

COMMENTS: Cholestyramine and colestipol dramatically reduce furosemide and thiazide absorption and diuretic effect. The effect of binding resins on other diuretics is not established, but it may be prudent to take the same precautions with them as well. The effect of **colesevelam** (Welchol) on diuretic absorption is not established; it may bind less tightly to other drugs than other binding resins do, but these diuretics appear to be particularly susceptible. **Ezetimibe** (Zetia) appears less likely to bind with other drugs than the binding resins.

CLASS 3: ASSESS RISK & TAKE ACTION IF NECESSARY
• *Circumvent/Minimize*: Minimize the interaction by giving the diuretic 2 hours before or 6 hours after the binding resin; keep a constant interval between diuretic and binding resin.
• *Monitor*: Monitor for altered diuretic response if binding resins are initiated, discontinued, or dose is changed, or if the interval between doses of the diuretic and binding resin is changed.

OBJECT DRUGS	PRECIPITANT DRUGS
Dofetilide (Tikosyn)	**Inhibitors of Cationic Tubular Secretion:** **Cimetidine** (Tagamet) **Dolutegravir** (Tivicay) **Ketoconazole** (Nizoral) **Triamterene** (Dyrenium) **Trimethoprim** (Bactrim, Septra)

COMMENTS: Approximately 70% of dofetilide is renally eliminated unchanged via active cationic secretion and glomerular filtration. Dofetilide-induced QTc prolongation increases with increasing plasma concentrations. Any drug known to compete for cationic secretion could result in an increase in dofetilide plasma concentration. Pending more study, other drugs reported to inhibit cationic tubular secretion (e.g., **amiodarone, procainamide, diltiazem, metformin,** and **verapamil**) should be used only with careful monitoring in patients taking dofetilide. **Verapamil** and **ketoconazole** also may inhibit the CYP3A4 metabolism of dofetilide.

CLASS 3: ASSESS RISK & TAKE ACTION IF NECESSARY
• *Consider Alternative*:
  Cimetidine: Other H_2-receptor antagonists such as **famotidine** (Pepcid), **nizatidine** (Axid), and **ranitidine** (Zantac) could be used instead of cimetidine.
  Triamterene: **Spironolactone** (Aldactone) or **amiloride** (Midamor) could be used as a potassium-sparing diuretic.
• *Monitor*: Patients taking dofetilide should be carefully monitored for increased QTc intervals if drugs that reduce its renal clearance are coadministered.

OBJECT DRUGS	PRECIPITANT DRUGS
Dolutegravir (Tivicay)	**Enzyme Inducers (UGT1A1):**
	Efavirenz (Sustiva)
	Etravirine (Intelence)
	Rifampin (Rifadin)
	St. John's wort
	Tipranavir (Aptivus)

COMMENTS: Dolutegravir is a substrate of UGT1A1. Inducers of UGT1A1 may reduce dolutegravir plasma concentrations by over 50%. Loss of antiviral activity may occur.

CLASS 3: ASSESS RISK & TAKE ACTION IF NECESSARY
* *Monitor*: If UGT1A1 inducers are coadministered with dolutegravir, consider increasing the dose of dolutegravir and monitor for reduced antiviral response.

OBJECT DRUGS	PRECIPITANT DRUGS
Dopamine Agonists:	**Dopamine Antagonists:**
Bromocriptine (Parlodel)	Haloperidol (Haldol)
Cabergoline (Dostinex)	Metoclopramide (Reglan)
Levodopa (Dopar)	Phenothiazines
Pramipexole (Mirapex)	Thiothixene (Navane)
Ropinirole (Requip)	

COMMENTS: Dopamine agonists, used for Parkinson's disease and other disorders, may be inhibited by dopamine antagonists resulting in a worsening of Parkinsonism. Conversely, the therapeutic effect of dopamine antagonists would be expected to be reduced by dopamine agonists.

CLASS 2: USE ONLY IF BENEFIT FELT TO OUTWEIGH RISK
* *Use Alternative*:
Antipsychotics: Atypical antipsychotics such as **clozapine** (Clozaril), **olanzapine** (Zyprexa), **quetiapine** (Seroquel), and **risperidone** (Risperdal) are less likely to produce extrapyramidal side effects. Theoretically, they would be less likely than butyrophenones, phenothiazines, or thioxanthines to inhibit dopamine agonists.
* *Monitor*: Be alert for a reduction in efficacy of both dopamine agonists and dopamine antagonists if they are coadministered.

OBJECT DRUGS	PRECIPITANT DRUGS	
Epinephrine (Systemic doses)	**Beta-blockers (Nonselective):**	
	Carteolol (Ocupress)	Pindolol (Visken)
	Carvedilol (Coreg)	Propranolol (Inderal)
	Levobunolol (Betagan)	Sotalol (Betapace)
	Nadolol (Corgard)	Timolol (Blocadren)
	Penbutolol (Levatol)	

COMMENTS: Non-cardioselective beta-blockers markedly increase the pressor response to epinephrine; this effect is not likely with epinephrine doses used for non-systemic effects (e.g., with local anesthetics) unless very large amounts are used. The increased blood pressure may be accompanied by bradycardia and cardiac arrhythmias. Patients prone to anaphylaxis should avoid all beta-blockers if possible (due to poor response to epinephrine should anaphylaxis occur). Ophthalmic use of beta-blockers can result in systemic beta-blockade in some patients.

CLASS 2: USE ONLY IF BENEFIT FELT TO OUTWEIGH RISK
* *Use Alternative*: Cardioselective beta-blockers are unlikely to result in hypertensive reactions in patients who receive systemic doses of epinephrine; thus, they are preferable to non-cardioselective beta-blockers if beta-blockers must be used. Cardioselective beta-blockers include **acebutolol** (Sectral), **atenolol** (Tenormin), **betaxolol** (Kerlone), **bisoprolol** (Zebeta), **esmolol** (Brevibloc), **metoprolol** (Lopressor), and **nebivolol** (Bystolic). Most cardioselective beta-blockers can become nonselective when used in large doses. Also, cardioselective agents that are metabolized by CYP2D6 such as metoprolol and nebivolol can become nonselective in people with reduced CYP2D6 activity, genetically or due to CYP2D6 inhibitors.

OBJECT DRUGS	PRECIPITANT DRUGS
Eplerenone (Inspra)	**Antimicrobials:**

Ciprofloxacin (Cipro)   **Posaconazole** (Noxafil)
Clarithromycin (Biaxin)   **Quinupristin** (Synercid)
Erythromycin (E-Mycin)   **Telithromycin** (Ketek)
Fluconazole (Diflucan)   **Troleandomycin** (TAO)
Itraconazole (Sporanox)   **Voriconazole** (Vfend)
Ketoconazole (Nizoral)

COMMENTS: Eplerenone is metabolized primarily by CYP3A4, and inhibitors of CYP3A4 may produce marked increases the serum levels of eplerenone. This may increase the risk of eplerenone toxicity, and the manufacturer states that eplerenone is contraindicated with potent CYP3A4 inhibitors.

CLASS 2: USE ONLY IF BENEFIT FELT TO OUTWEIGH RISK

- *Use Alternative*:
  Azole Antifungals: Itraconazole and ketoconazole are potent inhibitors of CYP3A4; fluconazole appears weaker, but in larger doses it also inhibits CYP3A4, and has been shown to produce moderate increases in plasma eplerenone concentrations. **Terbinafine** (Lamisil) does not appear to affect CYP3A4, and would not be expected to interact with eplerenone.
  Macrolide Antibiotics: Unlike erythromycin, clarithromycin and troleandomycin, **azithromycin** (Zithromax) and **dirithromycin*** do not appear to inhibit CYP3A4. (*not available in US)
  Telithromycin: The use of **azithromycin** (Zithromax) or a quinolone antibiotic other than ciprofloxacin should be considered.
- *Monitor*: If CYP3A4 inhibitors are used with eplerenone, monitor for excessive eplerenone effects such as hypotension and hyperkalemia; reduce eplerenone dose as needed.

OBJECT DRUGS	PRECIPITANT DRUGS
Eplerenone (Inspra)	**Antidepressants:** **Fluvoxamine** (Luvox) **Nefazodone**

COMMENTS: Eplerenone is metabolized primarily by CYP3A4, and potent inhibitors of CYP3A4 may produce marked increases the serum levels of eplerenone. This may increase the risk of eplerenone toxicity, and the manufacturer states that eplerenone is contraindicated with potent CYP3A4 inhibitors. Nefazodone is a potent CYP3A4 inhibitor, and fluvoxamine is a moderate inhibitor.

CLASS 2: USE ONLY IF BENEFIT FELT TO OUTWEIGH RISK

- *Use Alternative*: Sertraline (Zoloft), citalopram (Celexa), **escitalopram** (Lexapro), **venlafaxine** (Effexor), and **paroxetine** (Paxil) appear less likely to inhibit CYP3A4 than fluvoxamine. **Fluoxetine** (Prozac) appears to be a weak inhibitor of CYP3A4, but little is known about the effect of other antidepressants on eplerenone.
- *Monitor*: If CYP3A4 inhibitors are used with eplerenone, monitor for excessive eplerenone effects such as hypotension and hyperkalemia; reduce eplerenone dose as needed.

OBJECT DRUGS	PRECIPITANT DRUGS	
Eplerenone (Inspra)	**Enzyme Inhibitors:**	
	Amiodarone (Cordarone)	Diltiazem (Cardizem)
	Amprenavir (Agenerase)	Dronedarone (Multaq)
	Aprepitant (Emend)	Grapefruit
	Atazanavir (Reyataz)	Indinavir (Crixivan)
	Boceprevir (Victrelis)	Lomitapide (Juxtapid)
	Ceritinib (Zykadia)	Mifepristone (Korlym)
	Cobicistat (Stribild)	Nelfinavir (Viracept)
	Conivaptan (Vaprisol)	Ritonavir (Norvir)
	Cyclosporine (Neoral)	Saquinavir (Invirase)
	Darunavir (Prezista)	Telaprevir (Incivek)
	Delavirdine (Rescriptor)	Verapamil (Isoptin)

COMMENTS: Eplerenone is metabolized primarily by CYP3A4, and inhibitors of CYP3A4 may produce marked increases the serum levels of eplerenone. This may increase the risk of eplerenone toxicity, and the manufacturer states that eplerenone is contraindicated with potent CYP3A4 inhibitors. Aprepitant is a moderate inhibitor of CYP3A4, but is also likely to increase eplerenone concentrations.

CLASS 2: USE ONLY IF BENEFIT FELT TO OUTWEIGH RISK
* *Use Alternative*: Use an alternative to the enzyme inhibitor if possible.
  Calcium channel blockers: Calcium channel blockers other than diltiazem and verapamil are unlikely to inhibit CYP3A4.
  Grapefruit: Orange juice does not appear to inhibit CYP3A4.
* *Monitor*: If CYP3A4 inhibitors are used with eplerenone, monitor for excessive eplerenone effects such as hypotension and hyperkalemia; reduce eplerenone dose as needed.

OBJECT DRUGS	PRECIPITANT DRUGS
Ergot Alkaloids:	**Antidepressants:**
Dihydroergotamine (D.H.E. 45)	Fluvoxamine (Luvox)
Ergotamine (Cafergot)	Nefazodone
Methysergide (Sansert)	

COMMENTS: Ergotamine (and probably dihydroergotamine and methysergide) undergo first-pass metabolism by CYP3A4, and several reports of ergotism have appeared when CYP3A4 inhibitors were given concurrently. Fluvoxamine appears to be a modest CYP3A4 inhibitor but may produce increased ergotamine concentrations. Theoretically non-oral routes of ergot administration would interact much less than the oral route.

CLASS 2: USE ONLY IF BENEFIT FELT TO OUTWEIGH RISK
* *Use Alternative*: **Sertraline** (Zoloft), **citalopram** (Celexa), **escitalopram** (Lexapro), **venlafaxine** (Effexor), and **paroxetine** (Paxil) appear less likely to inhibit CYP3A4 than fluvoxamine. **Fluoxetine** (Prozac) appears to be a weak inhibitor of CYP3A4. Little is known about the effects of other antidepressants on ergot alkaloids.
* *Monitor*: If the combination is used, monitor carefully for evidence of ergotism such as ischemia of extremities (pain, tenderness, cyanosis, and low skin temperature), hypertension, and tongue ischemia.

OBJECT DRUGS	PRECIPITANT DRUGS	
Ergot Alkaloids:	**Antimicrobials:**	
Dihydroergotamine (D.H.E. 45)	**Ciprofloxacin** (Cipro)	**Posaconazole** (Noxafil)
Ergotamine (Cafergot)	**Clarithromycin** (Biaxin)	**Quinupristin** (Synercid)
Methysergide (Sansert)	**Erythromycin** (E-Mycin)	**Telithromycin** (Ketek)
	Fluconazole (Diflucan)	**Troleandomycin** (TAO)
	Itraconazole (Sporanox)	**Voriconazole** (Vfend)
	Ketoconazole (Nizoral)	

COMMENTS: Ergotamine (and probably dihydroergotamine and methysergide) undergo first-pass metabolism by CYP3A4, and several reports of ergotism have appeared when CYP3A4 inhibitors were given concurrently. Theoretically non-oral routes of ergot administration would interact much less than the oral route.

CLASS 2: USE ONLY IF BENEFIT FELT TO OUTWEIGH RISK
* *Use Alternative*:
  Azole Antifungals: Itraconazole and ketoconazole are potent inhibitors of CYP3A4; fluconazole appears weaker, but in larger doses it also inhibits CYP3A4. **Terbinafine** (Lamisil) does not appear to affect CYP3A4, and would not be expected to interact with ergot alkaloids.
  Macrolide Antibiotics: Unlike erythromycin, clarithromycin and troleandomycin, **azithromycin** (Zithromax) and **dirithromycin*** do not appear to inhibit CYP3A4. (*not available in US) Telithromycin: The use of **azithromycin** (Zithromax) or a quinolone antibiotic other than ciprofloxacin should be considered.
* *Monitor*: If the combination is used, monitor carefully for evidence of ergotism such as ischemia of extremities (pain, tenderness, cyanosis, and low skin temperature), hypertension, and tongue ischemia.

OBJECT DRUGS	PRECIPITANT DRUGS	
Ergot Alkaloids:	**Enzyme Inhibitors:**	
Dihydroergotamine (D.H.E. 45)	**Amiodarone** (Cordarone)	**Dronedarone** (Multaq)
Ergotamine (Cafergot)	**Amprenavir** (Agenerase)	**Grapefruit**
Methysergide (Sansert)	**Aprepitant** (Emend)	**Imatinib** (Gleevec)
	Atazanavir (Reyataz)	**Indinavir** (Crixivan)
	Boceprevir (Victrelis)	**Lapatinib** (Tykerb)
	Ceritinib (Zykadia)	**Lomitapide** (Juxtapid)
	Cobicistat (Stribild)	**Mifepristone** (Korlym)
	Conivaptan (Vaprisol)	**Nelfinavir** (Viracept)
	Cyclosporine (Neoral)	**Ritonavir** (Norvir)
	Darunavir (Prezista)	**Saquinavir** (Invirase)
	Delavirdine (Rescriptor)	**Telaprevir** (Incivek)
	Diltiazem (Cardizem)	**Verapamil** (Isoptin)

COMMENTS: Ergotamine (and probably dihydroergotamine and methysergide) undergo first-pass metabolism by CYP3A4, and several reports of ergotism have appeared when CYP3A4 inhibitors were given concurrently. Theoretically non-oral routes of ergot administration would interact much less than the oral route. Some of these combinations are listed as contraindicated in the product information (e.g., amprenavir or mifepristone with ergot alkaloids).

CLASS 2: USE ONLY IF BENEFIT FELT TO OUTWEIGH RISK
* *Use Alternative*: If possible, select an alternative to the CYP3A4 inhibitor for patients receiving concomitant ergot alkaloids.
  Calcium channel blockers: Calcium channel blockers other than diltiazem and verapamil are unlikely to inhibit the metabolism of ergot alkaloids.
  Grapefruit: Orange juice does not appear to inhibit CYP3A4.
* *Monitor*: If the combination is used, monitor carefully for evidence of ergotism such as ischemia of extremities (pain, tenderness, cyanosis, and low skin temperature), hypertension, and tongue ischemia.

OBJECT DRUGS	PRECIPITANT DRUGS
Ergot Alkaloids:	**Triptans:**
Dihydroergotamine (D.H.E. 45)	**Almotriptan** (Axert)
Ergotamine (Cafergot)	**Eletriptan** (Relpax)
Methysergide (Sansert)	**Frovatriptan** (Frova)
	Naratriptan (Amerge)
	Rizatriptan (Maxalt)
	Sumatriptan (Imitrex)
	Zolmitriptan (Zolmig)

COMMENTS: Theoretically, concurrent use of ergot alkaloids and triptans may result in excessive vasoconstriction. The manufactures of triptans state that concurrent use with ergot preparations is contraindicated.

CLASS 1: AVOID COMBINATION
• *Avoid*: Avoid use of triptans within 24 hours of ergot alkaloids.

OBJECT DRUGS	PRECIPITANT DRUGS	
HMG-CoA Reductase Inhibitors:	**Antimicrobials:**	
Atorvastatin (Lipitor)	**Ciprofloxacin** (Cipro)	**Posaconazole** (Noxafil)
Lovastatin (Mevacor)	**Clarithromycin** (Biaxin)	**Quinupristin** (Synercid)
Simvastatin (Zocor)	**Erythromycin** (E-Mycin)	**Telithromycin** (Ketek)
	Fluconazole (Diflucan)	**Troleandomycin** (TAO)
	Itraconazole (Sporanox)	**Voriconazole** (Vfend)
	Ketoconazole (Nizoral)	

COMMENTS: Lovastatin and simvastatin undergo extensive first-pass metabolism by CYP3A4; antimicrobials that inhibit CYP3A4 increase the risk of myopathy, rhabdomyolysis and acute renal failure. Most of the above CYP3A4 inhibitors are listed as contraindicated in the simvastatin product information (2013), and one would expect lovastatin to be just as likely as simvastatin to cause myopathy when combined with CYP3A4 inhibitors. Atorvastatin (Lipitor) undergoes less first-pass metabolism by CYP3A4 than lovastatin or simvastatin, so the risk of myopathy when combined with CYP3A4 inhibitors appears to be less. Nonetheless, some cases have been reported, including a fatal case of rhabdomyolysis possibly due to atorvastatin and fluconazole.

CLASS 2: USE ONLY IF BENEFIT FELT TO OUTWEIGH RISK
• *Use Alternative*:
  HMG-CoA Reductase Inhibitors: **Pravastatin** (Pravachol) is not metabolized by cytochrome P450 isozymes, but it appears to be an OATP substrate. Some of the above antimicrobials might affect OATP. Erythromycin substantially increases **pitavastatin** (Livalo) concentrations, possibly through inhibition of OATP. **Rosuvastatin** (Crestor) is also an OATP substrate, but erythromycin slightly *decreases* rosuvastatin plasma concentrations. **Fluvastatin** (Lescol) and **rosuvastatin** (Crestor) are metabolized by CYP2C9 and may interact with fluconazole and voriconazole.
  Azole Antifungals: Fluconazole appears to be a weaker inhibitor of CYP3A4 than itraconazole or ketoconazole. In larger doses it may inhibit CYP3A4 and should be used cautiously with lovastatin or simvastatin. Single doses of fluconazole would be unlikely to increase the risk of statin toxicity. **Terbinafine** (Lamisil) does not appear to inhibit CYP3A4.
  Macrolides: Unlike other macrolides, **azithromycin** (Zithromax) and **dirithromycin*** do not appear to inhibit CYP3A4 and would not be expected to interact with lovastatin or simvastatin. (*not available in US)
  Telithromycin: The use of azithromycin (Zithromax) or a quinolone antibiotic other than ciprofloxacin should be considered.
• *Circumvent/Minimize*: Consider discontinuing the statin during the antimicrobial, or reduce statin dose based on statin product information.
• *Monitor*: The patient should be alert for evidence of myopathy (muscle pain or weakness) and myoglobinuria (dark urine); CK concentrations are usually high.

OBJECT DRUGS	PRECIPITANT DRUGS
HMG-CoA Reductase Inhibitors:	**Calcium Channel Blockers:**
Atorvastatin (Lipitor)	Diltiazem (Cardizem)
Lovastatin (Mevacor)	Verapamil (Isoptin)
Simvastatin (Zocor)	

COMMENTS: Lovastatin and simvastatin undergo extensive first-pass metabolism by CYP3A4; calcium channel blockers that inhibit CYP3A4 (diltiazem and verapamil) increase the statin serum concentrations, increasing the risk of myopathy, rhabdomyolysis and acute renal failure. Consider the increased risk of myopathy against the specific need for one of the calcium channel blockers that inhibits CYP3A4. Atorvastatin (Lipitor) undergoes less first-pass metabolism by CYP3A4 than lovastatin or simvastatin, so the risk of myopathy when combined with CYP3A4 inhibitors appears to be less. Nonetheless, some cases have been reported.

CLASS 3: ASSESS RISK & TAKE ACTION IF NECESSARY
- *Consider Alternative*:
  HMG-CoA Reductase Inhibitors: **Pravastatin** (Pravachol) is not metabolized by cytochrome P450 isozymes, while **fluvastatin** (Lescol) and **rosuvastatin** (Crestor) are metabolized by CYP2C9—thus, they are not affected by CYP3A4 inhibition.
  Calcium channel blockers: Calcium channel blockers other than diltiazem and verapamil are unlikely to inhibit the metabolism of HMG-CoA reductase inhibitors. However, the 2013 product information for simvastatin states that **amlodipine** (Norvasc) may increase the risk of myopathy, and the simvastatin dose should not exceed 20 mg/day.
- *Circumvent/Minimize*: If the combination is used, consider reducing statin dose based on current statin product information.
- *Monitor*: If either diltiazem or verapamil is used with the statin, the patient should be alert for evidence of myopathy (muscle pain or weakness) or myoglobinuria (dark urine); CK concentrations are usually high.

OBJECT DRUGS	PRECIPITANT DRUGS
HMG-CoA Reductase Inhibitors:	**Fibrates:**
Atorvastatin (Lipitor)	Gemfibrozil (Lopid)
Lovastatin (Mevacor)	
Pitavastatin (Livalo)	
Rosuvastatin (Crestor)	
Simvastatin (Zocor)	

COMMENTS: Combined use of HMG-CoA reductase inhibitors and gemfibrozil may increase the risk of myopathy, which may lead to rhabdomyolysis and acute renal failure. There appear to be differences in the relative risk, depending upon which HMG-CoA is used. Only rare cases of myopathy have been reported with atorvastatin and gemfibrozil, but the risk appears somewhat higher when lovastatin or simvastatin are coadministered with gemfibrozil. Gemfibrozil has been shown to substantially increase the serum concentrations of simvastatin acid and lovastatin acid, while gemfibrozil tends to produce moderate elevations of rosuvastatin and pitavastatin plasma concentrations. The product information for some statins (eg, lovastatin and simvastatin) states that concurrent use of gemfibrozil is contraindicated.

CLASS 2: USE ONLY IF BENEFIT FELT TO OUTWEIGH RISK
- *Use Alternative*:
  HMG-CoA Reductase Inhibitors: Although definitive incidence data are not available, the risk of myopathy during concurrent **pravastatin** (Pravachol) or **fluvastatin** (Lescol) with gemfibrozil or fenofibrate appears to be minimal.
  Gemfibrozil: The risk of myopathy with combined use of statins and fenofibrate appears to be less than with gemfibrozil. For example, fenofibrate does not appear to have a pharmacokinetic interaction with simvastatin, and fenofibrate has little effect on pitavastatin or rosuvastatin plasma concentrations.
- *Circumvent/Minimize*: If the combination is used, consider reducing statin dose based on current statin product information.
- *Monitor*: If any HMG-CoA reductase inhibitor is used with gemfibrozil or another fibrate, the patient should be monitored for evidence of myopathy (muscle pain or weakness) and myoglobinuria (dark urine). Myopathy is usually associated with increased serum CK concentrations.

OBJECT DRUGS	PRECIPITANT DRUGS	
HMG-CoA Reductase Inhibitors:	**Enzyme Inhibitors:**	
Atorvastatin (Lipitor)	**Amiodarone** Cordarone)	**Fluvoxamine** (Luvox)
Lovastatin (Mevacor)	**Amprenavir** (Agenerase)	**Grapefruit**
Simvastatin (Zocor)	**Aprepitant** (Emend)	**Imatinib** (Gleevec)
	Atazanavir (Reyataz)	**Indinavir** (Crixivan)
	Boceprevir (Victrelis)	**Lomitapide** (Juxtapid)
	Ceritinib (Zykadia)	**Mifepristone** (Korlym)
	Cobicistat (Stribild)	**Nefazodone**
	Conivaptan (Vaprisol)	**Nelfinavir** (Viracept)
	Cyclosporine (Neoral)	**Ranolazine** (Ranexa)
	Danazol (Danocrine)	**Ritonavir** (Norvir)
	Darunavir (Prezista)	**Saquinavir** (Invirase)
	Delavirdine (Rescriptor)	**Telaprevir** (Incivek)
	Dronedarone (Multaq)	**Ticagrelor** (Brilinta)

COMMENTS: Lovastatin and simvastatin undergo extensive first-pass metabolism by CYP3A4; inhibitors of CYP3A4 increase the risk of myopathy, in some cases leading to rhabdomyolysis and acute renal failure. Some of these combinations (e.g., atazanavir + lovastatin or simvastatin) are listed as contraindicated in the product information. Atorvastatin (Lipitor) undergoes less first-pass metabolism by CYP3A4 than lovastatin or simvastatin, so the risk of myopathy when combined with CYP3A4 inhibitors appears to be less. Nonetheless, some cases have been reported. The mifepristone product information states that concurrent use of simvastatin or lovastatin is contraindicated. Ticagrelor is considered a weak CYP3A4 inhibitor, but it may increase simvastatin and simvastatin acid AUC by over 50%; atorvastatin was less affected by ticagrelor.

CLASS 2: USE ONLY IF BENEFIT FELT TO OUTWEIGH RISK
- *Use Alternative*:
  HMG-CoA Reductase Inhibitors: **Pravastatin** (Pravachol) is not metabolized by cytochrome P450 isozymes. **Fluvastatin** (Lescol) and **rosuvastatin** (Crestor) are metabolized by CYP2C9 and may not be affected by CYP3A4 inhibitors. Erythromycin, for example, slightly *decreased* the AUC of rosuvastatin. **Pitavastatin** (Livalo), pravastatin, and rosuvastatin all appear to be OATP substrates, and some of the above enzyme inhibitors might affect OATP. For example, erythromycin substantially increases pitavastatin concentrations, possibly through inhibition of OATP. [Note: Cyclosporine increases systemic exposure to *all* statins, although the risk of myopathy appears less with pravastatin.]
  Antidepressants: **Sertraline** (Zoloft), **citalopram** (Celexa), **venlafaxine** (Effexor), and **paroxetine** (Paxil) appear unlikely to inhibit CYP3A4, and **fluoxetine** (Prozac) appears to be a weak inhibitor of CYP3A4.
  Grapefruit: Orange juice does not appear to inhibit CYP3A4.
- *Circumvent/Minimize*: If CYP3A4 inhibitors are used, consider reducing statin dose based on current statin product information.
- *Monitor*: Patients receiving lovastatin, simvastatin or atorvastatin and a CYP3A4 enzyme inhibitor should be monitored for evidence of myopathy (muscle pain or weakness) and myoglobinuria (dark urine). Myopathy is usually associated with increased serum CK concentrations.

OBJECT DRUGS	PRECIPITANT DRUGS
HMG-CoA Reductase Inhibitors:	**OATP Inhibitors:**
Pitavastatin (Livalo)	**Cyclosporine** (Neoral)
Pravastatin (Pravachol)	**Eltrombopag** (Promacta)
Rosuvastatin (Crestor)	**Lopinavir** (Kaletra)
	Ritonavir (Norvir)

COMMENTS: Pitavastatin, pravastatin, and rosuvastatin are substrates for the transporter OATP, and inhibitors of OATP may increase the risk of myopathy. Combining pitavastatin with either ritonavir/lopinavir or cyclosporine is contraindicated in the pitavastatin product information. Some evidence suggests that lopinavir is a potent inhibitor of OATP1B1, which may be the mechanism for its ability to increase pitavastatin and rosuvastatin plasma concentrations. Eltrombopag has been shown to substantially increase rosuvastatin plasma concentrations, and it probably would affect pitavastatin and pravastatin as well.

CLASS 2: USE ONLY IF BENEFIT FELT TO OUTWEIGH RISK
- *Use Alternative*:
  HMG-CoA Reductase Inhibitors: Both cyclosporine and ritonavir/lopinavir are likely to increases systemic exposure to *all* statins, although the risk of myopathy may be less with **pravastatin** (Pravachol).
  Ritonavir/Lopinavir: The effect of other protease inhibitors on pitavastatin or rosuvastatin is not well studied. **Atazanavir** (Reyataz) may modestly increase pitavastatin plasma concentrations, and other protease inhibitors may also interact to varying degrees.
  Monitor: Patients receiving pitavastatin or rosuvastatin and an OATP inhibitor should be monitored for evidence of myopathy (muscle pain or weakness) and myoglobinuria (dark urine). Myopathy is usually associated with increased serum CK concentrations.

OBJECT DRUGS	PRECIPITANT DRUGS	
HMG-CoA Reductase Inhibitors:	**Enzyme Inducers:**	
Atorvastatin (Lipitor)	**Barbiturates**	**Nevirapine** (Viramune)
Lovastatin (Mevacor)	**Bosentan** (Tracleer)	**Oxcarbazepine** (Trileptal)
Simvastatin (Zocor)	**Carbamazepine** (Tegretol)	**Phenytoin** (Dilantin)
	Dabrafenib (Tafinlar)	**Primidone** (Mysoline)
	Dexamethasone (Decadron)	**Rifabutin** (Mycobutin)
	Efavirenz (Sustiva)	**Rifampin** (Rifadin)
	Etravirine (Intelence)	**Rifapentine** (Priftin)
	Lumacaftor (Orkambi)	**St. John's wort**

COMMENTS: Atorvastatin, lovastatin, and simvastatin are metabolized by CYP3A4 and enzyme inducers may substantially lower their serum concentrations. The magnitude of the effect may be sufficient to reduce the efficacy of the statin. For example, the potent inducer rifampin can lower simvastatin serum concentrations to less than 10% of normal, while even the modest enzyme inducer St. John's wort can lower simvastatin serum concentrations to about one-third of normal. Although little is known about the effects of enzyme inducers on **fluvastatin** (Lescol), it is metabolized primarily by CYP2C9 and is likely to interact with enzyme inducers as well. **Rosuvastatin** (Crestor) has minimal CYP2C9 metabolism and will be unlikely to be affected by enzyme inducers.

CLASS 3: ASSESS RISK & TAKE ACTION IF NECESSARY
- *Consider Alternative*: If possible, select an alternative to the CYP3A4 inducer for patients receiving concomitant atorvastatin, lovastatin, or simvastatin.
  HMG-CoA Reductase Inhibitors: **Pravastatin** (Pravachol) is not metabolized by cytochrome P450 isozymes, and theoretically would not be affected by enzyme induction. Nonetheless, there is conflicting evidence on the effect of rifampin on pravastatin, with both increases and decreases in plasma pravastatin being reported. Rifampin appears to modestly *increase* **pitavastatin** (Livalo) plasma concentrations, perhaps through inhibition of OATP1B1.
- *Monitor:* If atorvastatin, lovastatin, or simvastatin is used with an enzyme inducer, monitor for impairment of cholesterol-lowering effect. Keep in mind that enzyme induction is usually gradual and may take days to weeks for onset and offset, depending on the specific inducer.

OBJECT DRUGS	PRECIPITANT DRUGS	
Immunosuppressants:	**Enzyme Inducers:**	
Cyclosporine (Neoral)	Barbiturates	Oxcarbazepine (Trileptal)
Everolimus (Afinitor)	Bosentan (Tracleer)	Phenytoin (Dilantin)
Sirolimus (Rapamune)	Carbamazepine (Tegretol)	Primidone (Mysoline)
Tacrolimus (Prograf)	Dabrafenib (Tafinlar)	Rifabutin (Mycobutin)
	Dexamethasone (Decadron)	Rifampin (Rifadin)
	Efavirenz (Sustiva)	Rifapentine (Priftin)
	Etravirine (Intelence)	St. John's wort
	Lumacaftor (Orkambi)	
	Nevirapine (Viramune)	

COMMENTS: Enzyme inducers have been reported to enhance the metabolism of these immunosuppressants. This effect is probably due to induction of CYP3A4 and P-glycoprotein (PGP). Preliminary evidence suggests that levothyroxine acts as a PGP inducer in the small intestine; other thyroid hormones probably act similarly.

CLASS 2: USE ONLY IF BENEFIT FELT TO OUTWEIGH RISK
- *Use Alternative*: Use an alternative to the enzyme inducer if possible.
- *Monitor*: If an enzyme inducer is necessary, monitor for altered immunosuppressant effect if an enzyme inducer is initiated, discontinued, or changed in dosage; substantial dosage adjustments of immunosuppressants may be necessary. Keep in mind that enzyme induction is usually gradual and may take days to weeks for onset and offset, depending on the specific inducer.

OBJECT DRUGS	PRECIPITANT DRUGS	
Immunosuppressants:	**Antimicrobials:**	
Cyclosporine (Neoral)	Azithromycin (Zithromax)	Ketoconazole (Nizoral)
Everolimus (Afinitor)	Ciprofloxacin (Cipro)	Posaconazole (Noxafil)
Sirolimus (Rapamune)	Clarithromycin (Biaxin)	Quinupristin (Synercid)
Tacrolimus (Prograf)	Clotrimazole (Mycelex)	Telithromycin (Ketek)
	Erythromycin (E-Mycin)	Troleandomycin (TAO)
	Fluconazole (Diflucan)	Voriconazole (Vfend)
	Itraconazole (Sporanox)	

COMMENTS: These antimicrobial agents may inhibit the CYP3A4 metabolism of cyclosporine, sirolimus, and tacrolimus, thus increasing their effect and potential toxicity. Inhibition of P-glycoprotein (PGP) may also contribute to the interactions. Azithromycin does not inhibit CYP3A4, but appears to inhibit PGP; it may increase plasma concentrations of these immunosuppressants by this mechanism. Clotrimazole troches have been shown to elevate tacrolimus blood levels, and would also be expected to interact with cyclosporine and sirolimus. Some of these combinations are listed as contraindicated by the manufacturer (eg, sirolimus + voriconazole.)

CLASS 2: USE ONLY IF BENEFIT FELT TO OUTWEIGH RISK
- *Use Alternative*:
  Azole Antifungals: Itraconazole and ketoconazole are potent inhibitors of CYP3A4; fluconazole appears weaker, but in larger doses it also inhibits CYP3A4. **Terbinafine** (Lamisil) does not appear to affect CYP3A4, and would not be expected to interact with ergot alkaloids. In fact, terbinafine may slightly increase cyclosporine clearance according to the manufacturer.
  Macrolide Antibiotics: Consider using an alternative antibiotic.
  Telithromycin: Consider using an alternative antibiotic.
- *Monitor*: Monitor for altered immunosuppressant effect if a CYP3A4-inhibiting or PGP-inhibiting antimicrobial agent is initiated, discontinued, or changed in dosage. Substantial dosage reductions for the immunosuppressant may be needed in some cases.

OBJECT DRUGS	PRECIPITANT DRUGS	
Immunosuppressants:	**Enzyme Inhibitors:**	
Cyclosporine (Neoral)	**Amiodarone** (Cordarone)	**Diltiazem** (Cardizem)
Everolimus (Afinitor)	**Amprenavir** (Agenerase)	**Dronedarone** (Multaq)
Sirolimus (Rapamune)	**Androgens**	**Fluvoxamine** (Luvox)
Tacrolimus (Prograf)	**Aprepitant** (Emend)	**Grapefruit**
	Atazanavir (Reyataz)	**Indinavir** (Crixivan)
	Berberine (Goldenseal)	**Lomitapide** (Juxtapid)
	Boceprevir (Victrelis)	**Methoxsalen** (Oxsoralen)
	Ceritinib (Zykadia)	**Mifepristone** (Korlym)
	Chloroquine (Aralen)	**Nefazodone**
	Cobicistat (Stribild)	**Nelfinavir** (Viracept)
	Conivaptan (Vaprisol)	**Nicardipine** (Cardene)
	Contraceptives, Oral	**Ritonavir** (Norvir)
	Danazol (Danocrine)	**Saquinavir** (Invirase)
	Darunavir (Prezista)	**Telaprevir** (Incivek)
	Delavirdine (Rescriptor)	**Verapamil** (Isoptin)

COMMENTS: The enzyme inhibitors listed here may inhibit cyclosporine, sirolimus, and tacrolimus elimination via CYP3A4 and/or P-glycoprotein (PGP), thus potentially increasing immunosuppressant effect and toxicity. Oral contraceptives also appear to increase cyclosporine plasma levels, although the mechanism is not clear. Aprepitant is a CYP3A4 inhibitor, but it had only a small effect on intravenous tacrolimus; oral tacrolimus would probably be more affected. Methoxsalen produced modest increases in cyclosporine concentrations, but some subjects had substantial increases.

CLASS 2: USE ONLY IF BENEFIT FELT TO OUTWEIGH RISK
- *Use Alternative*: Use alternative to CYP3A4 inhibitor if possible.
  Antidepressants: **Sertraline** (Zoloft), **citalopram** (Celexa), **venlafaxine** (Effexor), and **paroxetine** (Paxil) appear less likely to inhibit CYP3A4 than fluvoxamine. **Fluoxetine** (Prozac) appears to be a weak inhibitor of CYP3A4.
  Calcium channel blockers: Calcium channel blockers other than diltiazem and verapamil are unlikely to inhibit CYP3A4.
  Grapefruit: Orange juice does not appear to inhibit CYP3A4.
- *Monitor*: If cyclosporine, sirolimus, or tacrolimus is initiated in the presence of CYP3A4 inhibitor therapy, it would be prudent to start with conservative doses of the immunosuppressant. Monitor for altered immunosuppressant effect if an enzyme inhibitor is initiated, discontinued, or changed in dosage. Substantial dosage reductions for the immunosuppressant may be needed in some cases.

OBJECT DRUGS	PRECIPITANT DRUGS	
Irinotecan (Camptosar)	**Enzyme Inducers:**	
	Barbiturates	**Phenytoin** (Dilantin)
	Carbamazepine (Tegretol)	**Primidone** (Mysoline)
	Dabrafenib (Tafinlar)	**Rifabutin** (Mycobutin)
	Dexamethasone (Decadron)	**Rifampin** (Rifadin)
	Efavirenz (Sustiva)	**Rifapentine** (Priftin)
	Lumacaftor (Orkambi)	**St. John's wort**
	Nevirapine (Viramune)	**Smoking**
	Oxcarbazepine (Trileptal)	

COMMENTS: Enzyme-inducers such as carbamazepine, phenobarbital, phenytoin, and St. John's wort have reduced serum concentrations of irinotecan and its active metabolite (SN-38), probably by increasing the CYP3A4 metabolism of irinotecan and the glucuronide conjugation of SN-38. In one study, cigarette smokers had almost 40% lower exposure to the active metabolite (SN-38) than non-smokers. Medicinal cannabis (given as a tea) did not affect irinotecan metabolism in another study.

CLASS 3: ASSESS RISK & TAKE ACTION IF NECESSARY
- *Consider Alternative*:

  Anticonvulsants: In patients on irinotecan it would be desirable to use anticonvulsants that are not enzyme inducers, but in many cases it may not be reasonable to change the patient's anticonvulsant regimen.

  HIV Medications. Since most antiviral medications are either inducers or inhibitors, it is probably best just to monitor patients and adjust irinotecan doses as needed.

  St. John's wort: Given the questionable benefit of St. John's wort, it would be prudent to avoid giving it with irinotecan.

- *Monitor*: Monitor for altered irinotecan effect if enzyme inducers are initiated, discontinued, or changed in dosage. Adjustments in irinotecan dosage may be necessary. Keep in mind that enzyme induction is usually gradual and may take days to weeks for onset and offset, depending on the specific inducer.

OBJECT DRUGS	PRECIPITANT DRUGS	
Irinotecan (Camptosar)	**Antimicrobials:**	
	Ciprofloxacin (Cipro)	**Posaconazole** (Noxafil)
	Clarithromycin (Biaxin)	**Quinupristin** (Synercid)
	Erythromycin (E-Mycin)	**Telithromycin** (Ketek)
	Fluconazole (Diflucan)	**Troleandomycin** (TAO)
	Itraconazole (Sporanox)	**Voriconazole** (Vfend)
	Ketoconazole (Nizoral)	

COMMENTS: CYP3A4 inhibitors may increase serum concentrations of irinotecan and its active metabolite (SN-38). Ketoconazole, for example, increased SN-38 AUC by 109%. Part of the effect of ketoconazole may be due to inhibition of the glucuronidation of SN-38 to SN-38G by UGT1A1, so it is not clear that all CYP3A4 inhibitors would necessarily interact with irinotecan. Nonetheless, the product information for irinotecan states that strong CYP3A4 inhibitors should not be used concurrently. It appears that SN-38G can be transformed back into SN-38 in the intestine by bacterial beta-glucuronidases, and be reabsorbed into the circulation. Thus, it is theoretically possible that some antibiotics could interfere with the enterohepatic circulation of irinotecan by killing these bacteria, thus tending to *reduce* irinotecan plasma concentrations.

CLASS 3: ASSESS RISK & TAKE ACTION IF NECESSARY
Consider Alternative:

Azole Antifungals: Fluconazole is usually a weaker inhibitor of CYP3A4 unless large doses are used. **Terbinafine** (Lamisil) does not appear to inhibit CYP3A4.

Macrolides: Unlike other macrolides, **azithromycin** (Zithromax) and **dirithromycin*** do not appear to inhibit CYP3A4 and would not be expected to interact with irinotecan. (*not available in US)

Telithromycin: The use of **azithromycin** (Zithromax) or a quinolone antibiotic other than ciprofloxacin should be considered.

OBJECT DRUGS	PRECIPITANT DRUGS	
Irinotecan (Camptosar)	**Enzyme Inhibitors:**	
	Amiodarone (Cordarone)	**Dronedarone** (Multaq)
	Amprenavir (Agenerase)	**Grapefruit**
	Aprepitant (Emend)	**Imatinib** (Gleevec)
	Atazanavir (Reyataz)	**Indinavir** (Crixivan)
	Boceprevir (Victrelis)	**Lapatinib** (Tykerb)
	Ceritinib (Zykadia)	**Lomitapide** (Juxtapid)
	Cobicistat (Stribild)	**Mifepristone** (Korlym)
	Conivaptan (Vaprisol)	**Nelfinavir** (Viracept)
	Cyclosporine (Neoral)	**Ritonavir** (Norvir)
	Darunavir (Prezista)	**Saquinavir** (Invirase)
	Delavirdine (Rescriptor)	**Telaprevir** (Incivek)
	Diltiazem (Cardizem)	**Verapamil** (Isoptin)

COMMENTS: CYP3A4 inhibitors may increase serum concentrations of irinotecan and its active metabolite (SN-38). Ketoconazole, for example, increased SN-38 AUC by 109%. Part of the effect of ketoconazole may be due to inhibition of the glucuronidation of SN-38 to SN-38G by UGT1A1, so it is not clear that all CYP3A4 inhibitors would necessarily interact with irinotecan. Nonetheless, the product information for irinotecan states that strong CYP3A4 inhibitors should not be used concurrently.

CLASS 3: ASSESS RISK & TAKE ACTION IF NECESSARY
- *Consider Alternative*:
  Calcium channel blockers: Calcium channel blockers other than diltiazem and verapamil are unlikely to inhibit the metabolism of irinotecan.
  Grapefruit: Orange juice does not appear to inhibit CYP3A4.
- *Monitor*: Monitor for altered irinotecan effect if CYP3A4 inhibitors are initiated, discontinued, or changed in dosage. Changes in irinotecan dosage may be necessary.

OBJECT DRUGS		PRECIPITANT DRUGS
Kinase Inhibitors:		**Antidepressants:**
Axitinib (Inlyta)	**Imatinib** (Gleevec)	**Fluvoxamine** (Luvox)
Bosutinib (Bosulif)	**Lapatinib** (Tykerb)	**Nefazodone**
Cabozantinib (Cometriq)	**Nilotinib** (Tasigna)	
Ceritinib (Zykadia)	**Osimertinib** (Tagrisso)	
Cobimetinib (Cotellic)	**Pazopanib** (Votrient)	
Crizotinib (Xalkori)	**Regorafenib** (Stivarga)	
Dabrafenib (Tafinlar)	**Ruxolitinib** (Jakafi)	
Dasatinib (Sprycel)	**Sorafenib** (Nexavar)	
Erlotinib (Tarceva)	**Sunitinib** (Sutent)	
Gefitinib (Iressa)	**Tofacitinib** (Xeljanz)	
Ibrutinib (Imbruvica)	**Vandetanib** (Caprelsa)	
Idelalisib (Zydelig)	**Vemurafenib** (Zelboraf)	

COMMENTS: Although data are limited, these antidepressants may increase the plasma levels of kinase inhibitors. Toxicity includes skin rashes, anemia, hemorrhage, and GI symptoms. Assume that all CYP3A4 inhibitors interact until proven otherwise.

CLASS 3: ASSESS RISK & TAKE ACTION IF NECESSARY
- *Consider Alternative*:
  Antidepressants: **Citalopram** (Celexa), **desvenlafaxine** (Pristiq), **paroxetine** (Paxil), **sertraline** (Zoloft), and **venlafaxine** (Effexor) appear to have minimal effects on CYP3A4. **Fluoxetine** (Prozac) appears to be a weak inhibitor of CYP3A4.
- *Monitor*: Monitor for altered antineoplastic response if the CYP3A4 inhibitor is initiated, discontinued, or changed in dosage.

OBJECT DRUGS		PRECIPITANT DRUGS
Kinase Inhibitors:		**Antimicrobials:**
Axitinib (Inlyta)	**Imatinib** (Gleevec)	**Ciprofloxacin** (Cipro)
Bosutinib (Bosulif)	**Lapatinib** (Tykerb)	**Clarithromycin** (Biaxin)
Cabozantinib (Cometriq)	**Nilotinib** (Tasigna)	**Erythromycin** (E-Mycin)
Ceritinib (Zykadia)	**Osimertinib** (Tagrisso)	**Fluconazole** (Diflucan)
Cobimetinib (Cotellic)	**Pazopanib** (Votrient)	**Isoniazid** (INH)
Crizotinib (Xalkori)	**Regorafenib** (Stivarga)	**Itraconazole** (Sporanox)
Dabrafenib (Tafinlar)	**Ruxolitinib** (Jakafi)	**Ketoconazole** (Nizoral)
Dasatinib (Sprycel)	**Sorafenib** (Nexavar)	**Posaconazole** (Noxafil)
Erlotinib (Tarceva)	**Sunitinib** (Sutent)	**Quinupristin** (Synercid)
Gefitinib (Iressa)	**Tofacitinib** (Xeljanz)	**Telithromycin** (Ketek)
Ibrutinib (Imbruvica)	**Vandetanib** (Caprelsa)	**Troleandomycin** (TAO)
Idelalisib (Zydelig)	**Vemurafenib** (Zelboraf)	**Voriconazole** (Vfend)

COMMENTS: Although data are limited, these antimicrobials may increase the plasma levels of kinase inhibitors. Toxicity includes skin rashes, anemia, hemorrhage, and GI symptoms. Assume that all CYP3A4 inhibitors interact until proven otherwise.

CLASS 3: ASSESS RISK & TAKE ACTION IF NECESSARY
- *Consider Alternative*:
  Azole Antifungals: Fluconazole is usually a weaker inhibitor of CYP3A4 unless large doses are used. **Terbinafine** (Lamisil) does not appear to affect CYP3A4.
  Macrolide Antibiotics: **Azithromycin** (Zithromax) does not appear to inhibit CYP3A4 and would be unlikely to interact.
- *Monitor*: Monitor for altered antineoplastic response if the CYP3A4 inhibitor is initiated, discontinued, or changed in dosage.

OBJECT DRUGS	PRECIPITANT DRUGS	
Kinase Inhibitors:	**Enzyme Inhibitors:**	
Axitinib (Inlyta)	Amiodarone (Cordarone)	**Grapefruit**
Bosutinib (Bosulif)	Amprenavir (Agenerase)	Indinavir (Crixivan)
Cabozantinib (Cometriq)	Aprepitant (Emend)	Lomitapide (Juxtapid)
Ceritinib (Zykadia)	Atazanavir (Reyataz)	Mifepristone (Korlym)
Cobimetinib (Cotellic)	Boceprevir (Victrelis)	Nelfinavir (Viracept)
Crizotinib (Xalkori)	Cobicistat (Stribild)	Ritonavir (Norvir)
Dabrafenib (Tafinlar)	Conivaptan (Vaprisol)	Saquinavir (Invirase)
Dasatinib (Sprycel)	Cyclosporine (Neoral)	Telaprevir (Incivek)
Erlotinib (Tarceva)	Darunavir (Prezista)	Verapamil (Isoptin)
Gefitinib (Iressa)	Delavirdine (Rescriptor)	
Ibrutinib (Imbruvica)	Diltiazem (Cardizem)	
Idelalisib (Zydelig)	Dronedarone (Multaq)	
Imatinib (Gleevec)		
Lapatinib (Tykerb)		
Nilotinib (Tasigna)		
Osimertinib (Tagrisso)		
Pazopanib (Votrient)		
Regorafenib (Stivarga)		
Ruxolitinib (Jakafi)		
Sorafenib (Nexavar)		
Sunitinib (Sutent)		
Tofacitinib (Xeljanz)		
Vandetanib (Caprelsa)		
Vemurafenib (Zelboraf)		

COMMENTS: Although data are limited, assume that all CYP3A4 inhibitors may increase the plasma levels of kinase inhibitors. Toxicity including skin rashes, anemia, hemorrhage, and gastrointestinal symptoms could result.

CLASS 3: ASSESS RISK & TAKE ACTION IF NECESSARY
* *Consider Alternative*:
    Calcium Channel Blockers: Calcium channel blockers other than diltiazem and verapamil are unlikely to inhibit the metabolism of these kinase inhibitors.
    Grapefruit: Orange juice does not appear to inhibit CYP3A4.
* *Monitor*: Monitor for altered antineoplastic response if the CYP3A4 inhibitor is initiated, discontinued, or changed in dosage.

OBJECT DRUGS		PRECIPITANT DRUGS
Kinase Inhibitors:		**Enzyme Inducers:**
Axitinib (Inlyta)	Lapatinib (Tykerb)	Barbiturates
Bosutinib (Bosulif)	Nilotinib (Tasigna)	Bosentan (Tracleer)
Cabozantinib (Cometriq)	Osimertinib (Tagrisso)	Carbamazepine (Tegretol)
Ceritinib (Zykadia)	Pazopanib (Votrient)	Dabrafenib (Tafinlar)
Cobimetinib (Cotellic)	Regorafenib (Stivarga)	Efavirenz (Sustiva)
Crizotinib (Xalkori)	Ruxolitinib (Jakafi)	Etravirine (Intelence)
Dabrafenib (Tafinlar)	Sorafenib (Nexavar)	Lumacaftor (Orkambi)
Dasatinib (Sprycel)	Sunitinib (Sutent)	Nevirapine (Viramune)
Erlotinib (Tarceva)	Tofacitinib (Xeljanz)	Oxcarbazepine (Trileptal)
Gefitinib (Iressa)	Vandetanib (Caprelsa)	Phenytoin (Dilantin)
Ibrutinib (Imbruvica)	Vemurafenib (Zelboraf)	Primidone (Mysoline)
Idelalisib (Zydelig)		Rifabutin (Mycobutin)
Imatinib (Gleevec)		Rifampin (Rifadin)
		Rifapentine (Priftin)
		St. John's wort

COMMENTS: Although data are limited, these enzyme inducers may decrease the plasma levels of kinase inhibitors. Reduction in the expected antineoplastic activity or resistance may occur. Lapatinib is metabolized into a hepatotoxic metabolite; inducers may increase the risk of hepatotoxicity.

CLASS 3: ASSESS RISK & TAKE ACTION IF NECESSARY
- *Monitor:* Monitor for altered antineoplastic response if the CYP3A4 inducer is initiated, discontinued, or changed in dosage.

OBJECT DRUGS	PRECIPITANT DRUGS	
Kinase Inhibitors:	**Gastric Antisecretory Agents:**	
Bosutinib (Bosulif)	**Cimetidine** (Tagamet)	**Nizatidine** (Axid)
Ceritinib (Zykadia)	**Dexlansoprazole** (Kapidex)	**Omeprazole** (Prilosec)
Dabrafenib (Tafinlar)	**Esomeprazole** (Nexium)	**Pantoprazole** (Protonix)
Dasatinib (Sprycel)	**Famotidine** (Pepcid)	**Rabeprazole** (Aciphex)
Erlotinib (Tarceva)	**Lansoprazole** (Prevacid)	**Ranitidine** (Zantac)
Gefitinib (Iressa)		
Lapatinib (Tykerb)		
Nilotinib (Tasigna)		
Pazopanib (Votrient)		
Sorafenib (Nexavar)		

COMMENTS: Several kinase inhibitors are dependent on an acidic gastric pH for dissolution. Administration with antisecretory agents that increase gastric pH will reduce the bioavailability of the kinase inhibitor. Antacids may also interact.

CLASS 3: ASSESS RISK & TAKE ACTION IF NECESSARY
- *Monitor:* Monitor for altered antineoplastic response if the gastric antisecretory agent is initiated, discontinued, or changed in dosage.

OBJECT DRUGS	PRECIPITANT DRUGS	
Lamotrigine (Lamictal)	**Enzyme Inducers:**	
	Barbiturates	**Phenytoin** (Dilantin)
	Carbamazepine (Tegretol)	**Primidone** (Mysoline)
	Dabrafenib (Tafinlar)	**Rifabutin** (Mycobutin)
	Efavirenz (Sustiva)	**Rifampin** (Rifadin)
	Nevirapine (Viramune)	**Rifapentine** (Priftin)
	Oxcarbazepine (Trileptal)	**St. John's wort**

COMMENTS: Enzyme-inducing drugs have been shown to reduce lamotrigine serum concentrations, probably by increasing lamotrigine glucuronidation. Some evidence suggests that lamotrigine may increase the risk of carbamazepine toxicity, but this has not been a consistent finding.

CLASS 3: ASSESS RISK & TAKE ACTION IF NECESSARY
- *Monitor:* Monitor for altered lamotrigine effect if enzyme inducers are initiated, discontinued, or changed in dosage. Adjustments in lamotrigine dosage may be necessary. Keep in mind that enzyme induction is usually gradual and may take days to weeks for onset and offset, depending on the specific inducer.

OBJECT DRUGS	PRECIPITANT DRUGS
Lamotrigine (Lamictal)	**Oral Contraceptives**

COMMENTS: Combined oral contraceptives have been shown in several studies to substantially reduce lamotrigine plasma concentrations; reduced lamotrigine efficacy may occur. The most likely mechanism is enhanced lamotrigine glucuronidation caused by the estrogen component, ethinyl estradiol.

CLASS 3: ASSESS RISK & TAKE ACTION IF NECESSARY
- *Consider Alternative*: Preliminary evidence suggests that progestogen-only contraceptives (regardless of method of administration) do not affect lamotrigine concentrations, but more study is needed. Many antiepileptic drugs interact with oral contraceptives by various mechanisms, so one must choose such combinations carefully.
- *Monitor*: If lamotrigine and oral contraceptives are used concurrently monitor for altered lamotrigine effect if an oral contraceptive is started, stopped, or if the patient is switched to a contraceptive product with a different hormone content.

OBJECT DRUGS	PRECIPITANT DRUGS
Lamotrigine (Lamictal)	Valproic Acid (Depakene)

COMMENTS: Valproic acid may substantially increase lamotrigine serum concentrations, probably through inhibition of lamotrigine metabolism. It has also been proposed that the combination of lamotrigine and valproic acid may increase the risk of serious skin eruptions such as Stevens-Johnson syndrome or toxic epidermal necrolysis, but a causal relationship has not been established. Isolated cases of hyperammonemic encephalopathy have been reported in patients receiving lamotrigine and valproic acid concurrently, but more study is needed to establish the clinical importance.

CLASS 3: ASSESS RISK & TAKE ACTION IF NECESSARY
- **Monitor:** Monitor for altered lamotrigine effect if valproic acid is initiated, discontinued, or changed in dosage. Adjustments in lamotrigine dosage may be necessary. Monitor also for evidence of encephalopathy (lethargy, tremor, asterixis, and elevated ammonia levels).

OBJECT DRUGS	PRECIPITANT DRUGS	
Lithium (Eskalith)	**ACE Inhibitors (ACEI):**	
	Benazepril (Lotensin)	Moexipril (Univasc)
	Captopril (Capoten)	Perindopril (Aceon)
	Enalapril (Vasotec)	Quinapril (Accupril)
	Fosinopril (Monopril)	Ramipril (Altace)
	Lisinopril (Prinivil)	Trandolapril (Mavik)

COMMENTS: Lithium toxicity has been reported when ACEI are used with lithium, although the magnitude of the effect is highly variable from patient to patient. The elderly appear to be at greater risk. The lithium toxicity can be severe, and there are many case reports of lithium toxicity following initiation of one of these drugs. In an epidemiologic study of elderly patients, ACEI were associated with a substantial increase in the risk of hospitalization due to lithium toxicity.

CLASS 3: ASSESS RISK & TAKE ACTION IF NECESSARY
- **Consider Alternative:** Depending on the indication for ACEI use, an alternate agent such as a calcium channel blocker could be considered. The use of an angiotensin receptor blocker (ARB) in place of the ACEI would not circumvent the interaction, since ARB also can cause lithium toxicity.
- **Monitor:** Monitor for altered lithium effects if ACEI are initiated, discontinued, changed in dosage, or if the patient is switched from one ACEI to another. Note that—depending on the original lithium serum concentration—it may take up to several weeks for lithium toxicity to become manifest. Lithium toxicity may cause nausea, vomiting, anorexia, diarrhea, slurred speech, confusion, lethargy, coarse tremor, and in severe cases can cause seizures, coma, and death.

OBJECT DRUGS	PRECIPITANT DRUGS	
Lithium (Eskalith)	**Angiotensin Receptor Blockers (ARBs):**	Losartan (Cozaar)
	Azilsartan (Edarbi)	Olmesartan (Benicar)
	Candesartan (Atacand)	Telmisartan (Micardis)
	Eprosartan (Teveten)	Valsartan (Diovan)
	Irbesartan (Avapro)	

COMMENTS: Lithium toxicity has been reported when ARBs are used with lithium, although the magnitude of the effect may be highly variable from patient to patient. The elderly appear to be at greater risk. The lithium toxicity can be severe, and there are case reports of lithium toxicity following initiation of one of these drugs.

CLASS 3: ASSESS RISK & TAKE ACTION IF NECESSARY
- **Consider Alternative:** Depending on the indication for ARB use, an alternate agent such as a calcium channel blocker could be considered. The use of an ACE inhibitor in place of ARBs would not circumvent the interaction, since ACE inhibitors also can cause lithium toxicity.
- **Monitor:** Monitor for altered lithium effects if these agents are initiated, discontinued, or changed in dosage. Note that—depending on the original lithium serum concentration—it may take up to several weeks for lithium toxicity to become manifest. Lithium toxicity may cause nausea, vomiting, anorexia, diarrhea, slurred speech, confusion, lethargy, coarse tremor, and in severe cases can cause seizures, coma, and death.

OBJECT DRUGS	PRECIPITANT DRUGS
Lithium (Eskalith)	**Loop Diuretics:**
	Bumetanide (Bumex)
	Ethacrynic Acid (Edecrin)
	Furosemide (Lasix)
	Torsemide (Demadex)

COMMENTS: Lithium toxicity has been reported when loop diuretics are used with lithium, although the magnitude of the effect may be variable from patient to patient. The elderly may be at greater risk. The lithium toxicity can be severe. In an epidemiologic study loop diuretics were associated with a substantial increase in the risk of hospitalization due to lithium toxicity.

CLASS 3: ASSESS RISK & TAKE ACTION IF NECESSARY
- *Monitor:* Monitor for altered lithium effects if loop diuretics are initiated, discontinued, or changed in dosage. Note that—depending on the original lithium serum concentration—it may take up to several weeks for lithium toxicity to become manifest. Lithium toxicity may cause nausea, vomiting, anorexia, diarrhea, slurred speech, confusion, lethargy, coarse tremor, and in severe cases can cause seizures, coma, and death.

OBJECT DRUGS	PRECIPITANT DRUGS	
Lithium (Eskalith)	**NSAIDs:**	
	Diclofenac (Voltaren)	Meclofenamate
	Diflunisal (Dolobid)	Mefenamic acid
	Etodolac (Lodine)	Meloxicam (Mobic)
	Fenoprofen (Nalfon)	Nabumetone (Relafen)
	Flurbiprofen (Ansaid)	Naproxen (Aleve)
	Ibuprofen (Motrin)	Oxaprozin (Daypro)
	Indomethacin (Indocin)	Piroxicam (Feldene)
	Ketoprofen (Orudis)	Sulindac (Clinoril)
	Ketorolac (Toradol)	Tolmetin (Tolectin)

COMMENTS: Lithium toxicity has been reported with concurrent NSAID therapy, although the magnitude of the effect is highly variable from patient to patient. The lithium toxicity can be severe, and there are many case reports of lithium toxicity following initiation of NSAIDs. In an epidemiologic study ACE inhibitors and loop diuretics were associated with a substantial increase in the risk of hospitalization due to lithium toxicity, but an association with thiazide diuretics and NSAIDs was not found. It may be that only predisposed patients develop lithium toxicity from NSAIDs; for example only some patients manifest substantial reductions in renal function following use of NSAIDs.

CLASS 3: ASSESS RISK & TAKE ACTION IF NECESSARY
- *Consider Alternative:* **Salicylates** do not appear to have much effect on plasma lithium concentrations and can be considered as alternatives to NSAIDs. **Sulindac** (Clinoril) appears less likely than other NSAIDs to increase lithium concentrations, but isolated cases have been reported. **Acetaminophen** is not likely to alter lithium elimination.
- *Monitor:* Monitor for altered lithium effects if NSAIDs are initiated, discontinued, changed in dosage, or if the patient is switched from one NSAID to another. Note that—depending on the original lithium serum concentration—it may take up to several weeks for lithium toxicity to become manifest. Lithium toxicity may cause nausea, vomiting, anorexia, diarrhea, slurred speech, confusion, lethargy, coarse tremor, and in severe cases can cause seizures and coma.

OBJECT DRUGS	PRECIPITANT DRUGS	
Lithium (Eskalith)	**Thiazide Diuretics:**	
	Bendroflumethiazide (Naturetin)	**Indapamide** (Lozol)*
	Benzthiazide (Exna)	**Methyclothiazide** (Enduron)
	Chlorothiazide (Diuril)	**Metolazone** (Zaroxolyn)*
	Chlorthalidone (Hygroton)*	**Polythiazide** (Renese)
	Hydrochlorothiazide (Hydrodiuril)	**Quinethazone** (Hydromox)*
	Hydroflumethiazide (Saluron)	**Trichlormethiazide** (Diurese)

Not strictly a thiazide, but has actions similar to the thiazide diuretics.

COMMENTS: Lithium toxicity has been reported with concurrent use of thiazide diuretics, although the magnitude of the effect is highly variable from patient to patient. The elderly may be at greater risk. In an epidemiologic study ACE inhibitors and loop diuretics were associated with a substantial increase in the risk of hospitalization due to lithium toxicity, but an association with thiazide diuretics and NSAIDs was not found. It may be that only predisposed patients develop lithium toxicity from thiazides.

CLASS 3: ASSESS RISK & TAKE ACTION IF NECESSARY
• *Monitor:* Monitor for altered lithium effects if thiazide diuretics are started, stopped, or changed in dosage. Depending on the original lithium serum concentration it may take up to several weeks for lithium toxicity to become manifest. Lithium toxicity may cause nausea, vomiting, anorexia, diarrhea, slurred speech, confusion, lethargy, coarse tremor, and in severe cases can cause seizures and coma.

OBJECT DRUGS	PRECIPITANT DRUGS	
Lomitapide (Juxtapid)	**Enzyme Inhibitors:**	
	Amiodarone (Cordarone)	**Dronedarone** (Multaq)
	Amprenavir (Agenerase)	**Fluvoxamine** (Luvox)
	Aprepitant (Emend)	**Grapefruit**
	Atazanavir (Reyataz)	**Indinavir** (Crixivan)
	Boceprevir (Victrelis)	**Mifepristone** (Korlym)
	Ceritinib (Zykadia)	**Nefazodone**
	Cobicistat (Stribild)	**Nelfinavir** (Viracept)
	Conivaptan (Vaprisol)	**Ritonavir** (Norvir)
	Cyclosporine (Neoral)	**Saquinavir** (Invirase)
	Darunavir (Prezista)	**Telaprevir** (Incivek)
	Delavirdine (Rescriptor)	

COMMENTS: Lomitapide is metabolized by CYP3A4, and inhibitors of CYP3A4 can produce dramatic increases in lomitapide plasma concentrations. For example, the strong CYP3A4 inhibitor, ketoconazole, produced a 27-fold increase in lomitapide AUC. Because increased lomitapide plasma levels can cause substantial toxicity, particularly hepatotoxicity, combining lomitapide with strong (or moderate) CYP3A4 inhibitors is considered contraindicated.

CLASS 1: AVOID COMBINATION
• *Avoid:* These enzyme inhibitors should not be given to patients receiving lomitapide due to the risk of serious hepatotoxicity and other toxic effects.
• *Use Alternative:* Use an alternative to the enzyme inhibitor if possible.
Antidepressants: **Sertraline** (Zoloft), **citalopram** (Celexa), **escitalopram** (Lexapro), **venlafaxine** (Effexor), and **paroxetine** (Paxil) appear less likely to inhibit CYP3A4. **Fluoxetine** (Prozac) appears to be only a weak inhibitor of CYP3A4.
Grapefruit: Orange juice does not appear to inhibit CYP3A4.

OBJECT DRUGS	PRECIPITANT DRUGS	
Lomitapide (Juxtapid)	**Antimicrobials:**	
	Ciprofloxacin (Cipro)	**Posaconazole** (Noxafil)
	Clarithromycin (Biaxin)	**Quinupristin** (Synercid)
	Erythromycin (E-Mycin)	**Telithromycin** (Ketek)
	Fluconazole (Diflucan)	**Troleandomycin** (TAO)
	Itraconazole (Sporanox)	**Voriconazole** (Vfend)
	Ketoconazole (Nizoral)	

COMMENTS: Lomitapide is metabolized by CYP3A4, and inhibitors of CYP3A4 can produce dramatic increases in lomitapide plasma concentrations. For example, the strong CYP3A4 inhibitor, ketoconazole, produced a 27-fold increase in lomitapide AUC. Because increased lomitapide plasma levels can cause substantial toxicity, particularly hepatotoxicity, combining lomitapide with strong (or moderate) CYP3A4 inhibitors is considered contraindicated.

CLASS 1: AVOID COMBINATION
- *Avoid*: These enzyme inhibitors should not be given to patients receiving lomitapide due to the risk of serious hepatotoxicity and other toxic effects.
- *Use Alternative*:
  Azole Antifungals: Itraconazole and ketoconazole are potent inhibitors of CYP3A4; fluconazole appears weaker, but in larger doses it also inhibits CYP3A4. **Terbinafine** (Lamisil) does not appear to affect CYP3A4, and would not be expected to interact with lomitapide.
  Macrolide Antibiotics: Unlike erythromycin, clarithromycin and troleandomycin, **azithromycin** (Zithromax) and **dirithromycin*** do not appear to inhibit CYP3A4. (*not available in US)
  Telithromycin: The use of **azithromycin** (Zithromax) or a quinolone antibiotic (other than ciprofloxacin) should be considered.

OBJECT DRUGS	PRECIPITANT DRUGS
Lomitapide (Juxtapid)	**Calcium Channel Blockers:**
	Diltiazem (Cardizem)
	Nicardipine (Cardene)
	Nifedipine (Procardia)
	Verapamil (Isoptin)

COMMENTS: Lomitapide is metabolized by CYP3A4, and calcium channel blockers that inhibit CYP3A4 are likely to produce substantial increases in lomitapide plasma concentrations. For example, the strong CYP3A4 inhibitor, ketoconazole, produced a 27-fold increase in lomitapide AUC. Because increased lomitapide plasma levels can cause substantial toxicity, particularly hepatotoxicity, combining lomitapide with strong (or moderate) CYP3A4 inhibitors is considered contraindicated. There is substantial evidence that diltiazem and verapamil inhibit CYP3A4, and some evidence that nicardipine and nifedipine inhibit CYP3A4; there is little evidence that other calcium channel blockers inhibit CYP3A4, although the product information for lomitapide suggests that amlodipine may inhibit lomitapide metabolism.

CLASS 1: AVOID COMBINATION
- *Avoid*: These calcium channel blockers should not be given to patients receiving lomitapide due to the risk of serious hepatotoxicity and other toxic effects.
- *Use Alternative*: Use an alternative to the enzyme inhibitor if possible.
  Calcium channel blockers: Calcium channel blockers other than diltiazem, nicardipine, nifedipine, and verapamil are less likely to inhibit the metabolism of lomitapide. Nonetheless, it would be prudent to monitor for lomitapide toxicity (i.e. hepatotoxicity) if any calcium channel blocker is given concurrently.

OBJECT DRUGS	PRECIPITANT DRUGS	
Lomitapide (Juxtapid)	**Enzyme Inhibitors:**	
	Alprazolam (Xanax)	**Fluoxetine** (Prozac)
	Bicalutamide (Casodex)	**Ranolazine** (Ranexa)
	Cilostazol (Pletal)	**Ticagrelor** (Brilinta)
	Cimetidine (Tagamet)	**Zileuton** (Zyflo)
	Contraceptives, Oral	

COMMENTS: Lomitapide is metabolized by CYP3A4, and even these "weak" inhibitors of CYP3A4 can produce increases in lomitapide plasma concentrations. For example oral contraceptives (considered weak CYP3A4 inhibitors) produced about a doubling of lomitapide exposure. Because increased lomitapide plasma levels can cause substantial toxicity, particularly hepatotoxicity, combining lomitapide with weak CYP3A4 inhibitors may require a reduction in lomitapide dosage.

CLASS 3: ASSESS RISK & TAKE ACTION IF NECESSARY
- *Circumvent/Minimize:* It would be prudent to limit lomitapide dosage to 30 mg/day in patients also taking any of these "weak" CYP3A4 inhibitors.
- *Consider Alternative*:
  Cimetidine: **Famotidine** (Pepcid), **nizatidine** (Axid), and **ranitidine** (Zantac) are unlikely to affect CYP3A4 activity, even though the lomitapide product information suggests that ranitidine is a weak CYP3A4 inhibitor.
  Antidepressants: **Sertraline** (Zoloft), **citalopram** (Celexa), **escitalopram** (Lexapro), **venlafaxine** (Effexor), and **paroxetine** (Paxil) appear less likely to inhibit CYP3A4.
- *Monitor:* If these combinations are used, monitor for evidence of lomitapide toxicity (eg, hepatotoxicity).

OBJECT DRUGS	PRECIPITANT DRUGS
MAO Inhibitors (nonselective):	**Antidepressants, Tricyclic:**
Furazolidone (Furoxone)	**Clomipramine** (Anafranil)
Isocarboxazid	**Imipramine** (Tofranil)
Methylene Blue	
Phenelzine (Nardil)	
Tranylcypromine (Parnate)	

COMMENTS: Nonselective MAO inhibitors (MAOI) may produce serotonin syndrome when combined with tricyclic antidepressants (TCAs), especially TCAs with substantial serotonergic effects such as clomipramine and imipramine. Nonselective MAOI and TCAs have been used safely with careful monitoring in experienced hands, but serotonin syndrome can be life-threatening.

CLASS 1: AVOID COMBINATION
- *Avoid:* Avoid clomipramine and imipramine in patients receiving nonselective MAOI. Avoiding **amitriptyline, doxepin,** and **desipramine** would also be prudent although the risk is probably less. At least 14 days (preferably 18-20 days) should elapse after stopping an MAOI before starting clomipramine or imipramine. If a TCA is to be used, use those with less serotonergic effects and monitor for evidence of serotonin syndrome (myoclonus, rigidity, tremor, hyperreflexia, fever, sweating, seizures, confusion, agitation, incoordination, and coma).

OBJECT DRUGS	PRECIPITANT DRUGS	
MAO Inhibitors (nonselective):	**Serotonergic Drugs:**	
Furazolidone (Furoxone)	**Bupropion** (Wellbutrin)	**Levomilnacipran** (Fetzima)
Isocarboxazid	**Citalopram** (Celexa)	**Milnacipran** (Savella)
Methylene Blue	**Cyclobenzaprine** (Flexeril)	**Paroxetine** (Paxil)
Phenelzine (Nardil)	**Desvenlafaxine** (Pristiq)	**Propoxyphene***
Tranylcypromine (Parnate)	**Dextromethorphan**	**Sertraline** (Zoloft)
	Duloxetine (Cymbalta)	**Tapentadol** (Nucynta)
	Escitalopram (Lexapro)	**Tetrabenazine** (Xenazine)
	Fentanyl (Sublimaze)	**Tramadol** (Ultram)
	Fluoxetine (Prozac)	**Trazodone** (Desyrel)
	Fluvoxamine (Luvox)	**Venlafaxine** (Effexor)
	Levomilnacipran (Fetzima)	**Vilazodone** (Viibryd)
	Meperidine (Demerol)	**Vortioxetine** (Brintellix)
	Methadone (Dolophine)	

* Propoxyphene (Darvon) was withdrawn from the US market.

COMMENTS: Nonselective MAO inhibitors (MAOI) may produce serotonin syndrome when combined with serotonergic drugs. Serotonin syndrome can be life-threatening. [Note: Concurrent use of 2 or more serotonergic drugs (from the 2 right columns above) may increase the risk of serotonin syndrome, but only isolated cases have been reported.] Bupropion is not generally considered a serotonergic drug, but purportedly may increase MAO inhibitor toxicity; the combination is considered contraindicated in the product information.

CLASS 1: AVOID COMBINATION
- *Avoid*: Avoid serotonergic drugs in patients receiving MAOI. At least 14 days (preferably 18-20 days) should elapse after stopping an MAOI before starting a serotonergic drug. At least 5 weeks should elapse after stopping **fluoxetine** before starting an MAOI. If such combinations are used, monitor for evidence of serotonin syndrome (myoclonus, rigidity, tremor, hyperreflexia, fever, sweating, seizures, confusion, agitation, incoordination, and coma).

OBJECT DRUGS	PRECIPITANT DRUGS	
MAO Inhibitors (nonselective):	**Sympathomimetics:**	
Furazolidone (Furoxone)	**Amphetamines**	**Metaraminol** (Aramine)
Isocarboxazid	**Atomoxetine** (Strattera)	**Methylphenidate** (Ritalin)
Methylene Blue	**Cocaine**	**Phendimetrazine** (Bontril)
Phenelzine (Nardil)	**Diethylpropion** (Tenuate)	**Phentermine** (Ionamin)
Tranylcypromine (Parnate)	**Dopamine**	**Phenylephrine**
	Ephedrine	**Pseudoephedrine** (Sudafed)
	Isometheptene (Midrin)	**Tapentadol** (Nucynta)
	Mazindol (Sanorex)	

COMMENTS: Indirect acting sympathomimetics result in release of the increased stores of norepinephrine, and may result in severe hypertension, hyperpyrexia, seizures, arrhythmias and death in patients on nonselective MAO inhibitors (MAOI). Direct acting sympathomimetics such as **epinephrine, isoproterenol** and **norepinephrine** do not appear to interact as much, because they do not cause release of norepinephrine. Nonetheless, one should still be alert for increased pressor effects. Phenylephrine is a direct acting sympathomimetic, but it can also cause hypertensive reactions in patients on nonselective MAOI, because it is a substrate for intestinal and hepatic MAOI.

CLASS 1: AVOID COMBINATION
- *Avoid*: Avoid the sympathomimetics for at least 14 days (preferably 18-20 days) after stopping an MAOI.

OBJECT DRUGS	PRECIPITANT DRUGS
MAO Inhibitors (nonselective):	**Antidepressants, Tricyclic:**
Linezolid (Zyvox)	Clomipramine (Anafranil)
MAO-B Inhibitors:	Imipramine (Tofranil)
Rasagiline (Azilect)	
Selegiline (Eldepryl)	

COMMENTS: Linezolid appears to be a weak MAOI, but serotonin syndrome has been reported when it is combined with serotonergic agents such as clomipramine and imipramine. Selective MAO-B inhibitors theoretically should not interact with TCAs, but in some patients MAO-B inhibitors may become nonselective thus increasing the risk of serotonin syndrome. Rasagiline is metabolized by CYP1A2 so theoretically, patients on CYP1A2 inhibitors may be more likely to develop nonselective MAO inhibition due to rasagiline. (For a list of CYP1A2 inhibitors, see CYP450 Table.)

CLASS 2: USE ONLY IF BENEFIT FELT TO OUTWEIGH RISK
- *Use Alternative:*
  Antidepressants: If a TCA is given to patients on linezolid or MAO-B inhibitors, use a TCA other than clomipramine or imipramine. Avoiding amitriptyline, doxepin and desipramine would also be prudent.
  Linezolid: **Tedizolid** (Sivextro) does not appear to be a MAOI to a clinically important degree, so is unlikely to increase the risk of serotonin syndrome. Also, depending on the antibiogram, one could consider alternative antibiotics such as **vancomycin** or **telavancin** (Vibativ) for linezolid.
- *Monitor:* If any TCA is used with linezolid or an MAO-B inhibitor, monitor for evidence of serotonin syndrome (myoclonus, rigidity, tremor, hyperreflexia, fever, sweating, seizures, confusion, agitation, incoordination, and coma).

OBJECT DRUGS	PRECIPITANT DRUGS	
MAO Inhibitors (nonselective):	**Serotonergic Drugs:**	
Linezolid (Zyvox)	Citalopram (Celexa)	Milnacipran (Savella)
MAO-B Inhibitors:	Cyclobenzaprine (Flexeril)	Paroxetine (Paxil)
Rasagiline (Azilect)	Desvenlafaxine (Pristiq)	Propoxyphene*
Selegiline (Eldepryl)	Dextromethorphan	Sertraline (Zoloft)
	Duloxetine (Cymbalta)	Tapentadol (Nucynta)
	Escitalopram (Lexapro)	Tetrabenazine (Xenazine)
	Fentanyl (Sublimaze)	Tramadol (Ultram)
	Fluoxetine (Prozac)	Trazodone (Desyrel)
	Fluvoxamine (Luvox)	Venlafaxine (Effexor)
	Meperidine (Demerol)	Vilazodone (Viibryd)
	Methadone (Dolophine)	Vortioxetine (Brintellix)
	Levomilnacipran (Fetzima)	

* Propoxyphene (Darvon) was withdrawn from the US market.

COMMENTS: Linezolid appears to be a weak MAOI, but serotonin syndrome has been reported when it is combined with serotonergic agents, including SSRIs and SNRIs. Selective MAO-B inhibitors theoretically should not interact with serotonergic drugs, and many patients have received these combinations safely. For example, one study found no interaction when rasagiline and citalopram were given together. Some patients on MAO-B inhibitors, however, may develop nonselective MAO inhibition. Rasagiline is metabolized by CYP1A2, so theoretically, patients on CYP1A2 inhibitors may be more likely to develop nonselective MAO inhibition due to rasagiline. (For a list of CYP1A2 inhibitors, see CYP 450 Table at front of book.) (Note: Concurrent use of 2 or more serotonergic drugs (from the 2 right columns above) may increase the risk of serotonin syndrome, but only isolated cases have been reported.)

CLASS 2: USE ONLY IF BENEFIT FELT TO OUTWEIGH RISK
- *Use Alternative:*
  Serotonergic Drug: If possible use an alternative to the serotonergic drug in patients on linezolid or MAO-B inhibitors. Note that some of these combinations may be listed as contraindicated in the product information.
  Linezolid: **Tedizolid** (Sivextro) does not appear to be a MAOI to a clinically important degree, so is unlikely to increase the risk of serotonin syndrome. Also, depending on the antibiogram, one could consider alternative antibiotics such as **vancomycin** or **telavancin** (Vibativ) for linezolid.

- *Monitor*: If serotonergic drugs are used with linezolid or MAO-B inhibitors, monitor for evidence of serotonin syndrome (myoclonus, rigidity, tremor, hyperreflexia, fever, sweating, seizures, confusion, agitation, incoordination, and coma).

OBJECT DRUGS	PRECIPITANT DRUGS	
MAO Inhibitors (nonselective):	**Sympathomimetics:**	
Linezolid (Zyvox)	**Amphetamines**	**Metaraminol** (Aramine)
MAO-B Inhibitors:	**Atomoxetine** (Strattera)	**Methylphenidate** (Ritalin)
Rasagiline (Azilect)	**Cocaine**	**Phendimetrazine** (Bontril)
Selegiline (Eldepryl)	**Diethylpropion** (Tenuate)	**Phentermine** (Ionamin)
	Dopamine	**Phenylephrine**
	Ephedrine	**Pseudoephedrine** (Sudafed)
	Isometheptene (Midrin)	**Tapentadol** (Nucynta)
	Mazindol (Sanorex)	

COMMENTS: Linezolid is a mild MAO inhibitor, but can produce (usually modest) increases in the pressor response to indirect-acting sympathomimetics such as pseudoephedrine. MAO-B inhibitors theoretically would be unlikely to interact, but some patients on these drugs may develop nonselective MAO inhibition. Rasagiline is metabolized by CYP1A2, so theoretically, patients on CYP1A2 inhibitors may be more likely to develop nonselective MAO inhibition due to rasagiline. (For a list of CYP1A2 inhibitors, see CYP 450 Table at front of book.) Direct acting sympathomimetics such as **epinephrine, isoproterenol** and **norepinephrine** do not appear to interact as much with MAO inhibitors, but one should still be alert for increased pressor effects.

CLASS 2: USE ONLY IF BENEFIT FELT TO OUTWEIGH RISK

- *Use Alternative*:
Linezolid: **Tedizolid** (Sivextro) does not appear to be a MAOI to a clinically important degree, so is unlikely to increase the risk of serotonin syndrome. Also, depending on the antibiogram, one could consider alternative antibiotics such as **vancomycin** or **telavancin** (Vibativ) for linezolid.
- *Monitor*: If sympathomimetic drugs are used with linezolid or MAO-B inhibitors, monitor for evidence of hypertension, fever, seizures, or arrhythmias; discontinue the sympathomimetic immediately if any of these findings are present.

OBJECT DRUGS	PRECIPITANT DRUGS	
Methotrexate	**Inhibitors of Anionic Tubular Secretion:**	
(Anticancer Doses)	**Ciprofloxacin** (Cipro)	**Probenecid** (Benemid)
Pralatrexate (Folotyn)	**Co-trimoxazole** (Septra)	**Thiazide Diuretics**

COMMENTS: In patients receiving antineoplastic doses of methotrexate, ciprofloxacin and co-trimoxazole have been associated with methotrexate toxicity such as bone marrow suppression and GI toxicity. A causal relationship is not well established, but the severity of the reactions dictates caution. The risk with low-dose methotrexate (e.g., for arthritis) is probably much lower, but one should still be alert for evidence of methotrexate toxicity. Probenecid can increase methotrexate levels by 2-3 fold. The effect of quinolones other than ciprofloxacin on methotrexate is not established, but be alert for evidence of methotrexate toxicity. Pralatrexate concentrations are increased by probenecid; caution with other inhibitors of renal clearance is warranted.

CLASS 2: USE ONLY IF BENEFIT FELT TO OUTWEIGH RISK

- *Monitor*: Monitor for altered methotrexate or pralatrexate effect if a renal tubular secretion inhibitor is initiated, discontinued, or changed in dose.

OBJECT DRUGS	PRECIPITANT DRUGS	
Methotrexate (Anticancer Doses) Pralatrexate (Folotyn)	**NSAIDs:**	
	Diclofenac (Voltaren)	Mefenamic acid
	Diflunisal (Dolobid)	Meloxicam (Mobic)
	Etodolac (Lodine)	Nabumetone (Relafen)
	Fenoprofen (Nalfon)	Naproxen (Aleve)
	Flurbiprofen (Ansaid)	Oxaprozin (Daypro)
	Ibuprofen (Motrin)	Piroxicam (Feldene)
	Indomethacin (Indocin)	Salicylates
	Ketoprofen (Orudis)	Sulindac (Clinoril)
	Ketorolac (Toradol)	Tolmetin (Tolectin)
	Meclofenamate	

COMMENTS: In patients receiving antineoplastic doses of methotrexate, NSAIDs and full dose salicylates have been associated with methotrexate toxicity such as bone marrow suppression and GI toxicity. The risk with low-dose methotrexate (e.g., for rheumatoid arthritis) is probably much lower; indeed, NSAIDs are often used with low-dose methotrexate in this situation. Nonetheless, one should still be alert for evidence of methotrexate toxicity. A Cochrane systematic review of studies involving patients on methotrexate *for arthritis* found that although NSAIDs did not appear to increase the risk of methotrexate toxicity, anti-inflammatory doses of aspirin combined with methotrexate may increase the risk of hepatic and renal malfunction. Pralatrexate concentrations are increased by probenecid, so caution with other potential inhibitors of renal clearance (such as NSAIDs) is warranted.

CLASS 2: USE ONLY IF BENEFIT FELT TO OUTWEIGH RISK

- *Use Alternative:* Consider **acetaminophen** instead of NSAIDs or salicylates. Preliminary evidence suggests that **celecoxib** (Celebrex) does not affect methotrexate pharmacokinetics and could be considered as an alternative. **Valdecoxib** (withdrawn from US market), however, may increase methotrexate serum concentrations.
- *Monitor:* Monitor for altered methotrexate or pralatrexate effect if a renal tubular secretion inhibitor is initiated, discontinued, or changed in dose.

OBJECT DRUGS	PRECIPITANT DRUGS	
Methotrexate (Anticancer Doses) Pralatrexate (Folotyn)	**Penicillins:**	
	Amoxicillin (Amoxil)	Oxacillin (Bactocill)
	Carbenicillin (Geocillin)	Piperacillin (Pipracil)
	Mezlocillin (Mezlin)	

COMMENTS: In patients receiving antineoplastic doses of methotrexate penicillins such as amoxicillin, carbenicillin, mezlocillin, oxacillin, and piperacillin have been associated with methotrexate toxicity such as bone marrow suppression and GI toxicity. A causal relationship is not well established, but the severity of the reactions dictates caution. The effect of other penicillins is not established, but one should be alert for evidence of methotrexate toxicity if any penicillin is given (especially if large doses are used). The risk with low-dose methotrexate (e.g., for arthritis) is probably much lower, but one should still be alert for evidence of methotrexate toxicity. Pralatrexate concentrations are increased by probenecid; caution with other inhibitors of renal clearance such as penicillins is warranted.

CLASS 2: USE ONLY IF BENEFIT FELT TO OUTWEIGH RISK

- *Monitor:* Monitor for altered methotrexate or pralatrexate effect if a renal tubular secretion inhibitor is initiated, discontinued, or changed in dose.

OBJECT DRUGS	PRECIPITANT DRUGS	
Methotrexate (Anticancer doses) Pralatrexate (Folotyn)	**Proton Pump Inhibitors:**	
	Dexlansoprazole (Dexilant)	Omeprazole (Prilosec)
	Esomeprazole (Nexium)	Pantoprazole (Protonix)
	Lansoprazole (Prevacid)	Rabeprazole (Aciphex)

COMMENTS: In patients receiving antineoplastic doses of methotrexate, several proton pump inhibitors (PPIs) have been associated with methotrexate toxicity such as bone marrow suppression and GI toxicity. The risk with low-dose methotrexate (e.g., for arthritis) is probably much lower, but one should still be alert for evidence of methotrexate toxicity. Although there is limited information on potential interactions of pralatrexate with PPIs, one should assume that it may interact as well until clinical evidence is available.

CLASS 2: USE ONLY IF BENEFIT FELT TO OUTWEIGH RISK

- *Use Alternative*: H_2-receptor antagonists are not known to interact with methotrexate, and may be safer alternatives to PPIs. Nonetheless, one should still monitor for altered methotrexate or pralatrexate effect if H_2-receptor antagonists are used.
- *Monitor*: Monitor for altered methotrexate or pralatrexate effect if a renal tubular secretion inhibitor is initiated, discontinued, or changed in dose.

OBJECT DRUGS	PRECIPITANT DRUGS	
Metoclopramide (Reglan)	**Enzyme Inhibitors:**	
	Abiraterone (Zytiga)	**Propafenone** (Rythmol)
	Amiodarone (Cordarone)	**Propoxyphene***
	Cimetidine (Tagamet)	**Quinidine** (Quinidex)
	Cinacalcet (Sensipar)	**Ritonavir** (Norvir)
	Clobazam (Onfi)	**Terbinafine** (Lamisil)
	Diphenhydramine (Benadryl)	**Thioridazine** (Mellaril)
	Haloperidol (Haldol)	
	Mirabegron (Myrbetriq)	

* Propoxyphene (Darvon) was withdrawn from the US market.

COMMENTS: Inhibitors of CYP2D6 prevent the metabolism of metoclopramide. Accumulation of metoclopramide may increase the risk of tardive dyskinesia and other movement disorders. Patients with renal disease may be at increased risk.

CLASS 3: ASSESS RISK & TAKE ACTION IF NECESSARY
- *Monitor:* Monitor for movement disorders if metoclopramide is administered with a CYP2D6 inhibitor.

OBJECT DRUGS	PRECIPITANT DRUGS	
Mifepristone (Korlym)	**Enzyme Inducers:**	
	Barbiturates	**Oxcarbazepine** (Trileptal)
	Bosentan (Tracleer)	**Phenytoin** (Dilantin)
	Carbamazepine (Tegretol)	**Primidone** (Mysoline)
	Dabrafenib (Tafinlar)	**Rifabutin** (Mycobutin)
	Dexamethasone (Decadron)	**Rifampin** (Rifadin)
	Efavirenz (Sustiva)	**Rifapentine** (Priftin)
	Lumacaftor (Orkambi)	**St. John's wort**
	Nevirapine (Viramune)	**Smoking**

COMMENTS: Mifepristone is metabolized by CYP3A4, and enzyme inducers may reduce serum concentrations of mifepristone. The product information for mifepristone states that enzyme inducers should not be administered with mifepristone therapy.

CLASS 2: USE ONLY IF BENEFIT FELT TO OUTWEIGH RISK
- *Use Alternative*:
  Anticonvulsants: In patients on mifepristone it would be desirable to use anticonvulsants that are not enzyme inducers, but in many cases it may not be reasonable to change the patient's anticonvulsant regimen.
  HIV Medications. Since most antiviral medications are either inducers or inhibitors, it is probably best just to monitor patients and adjust mifepristone doses as needed.
  St. John's wort: Given the questionable benefit of St. John's wort, it would be prudent to avoid giving it with mifepristone.
- *Monitor*: Monitor for altered mifepristone effect if enzyme inducers are initiated, discontinued, or changed in dosage. Adjustments in mifepristone dosage may be necessary. Keep in mind that enzyme induction is usually gradual and may take days to weeks for onset and offset, depending on the specific inducer.

OBJECT DRUGS	PRECIPITANT DRUGS	
Mifepristone (Korlym)	**Antimicrobials:**	
	Ciprofloxacin (Cipro)	Posaconazole (Noxafil)
	Clarithromycin (Biaxin)	Quinupristin (Synercid)
	Erythromycin (E-Mycin)	Telithromycin (Ketek)
	Fluconazole (Diflucan)	Troleandomycin (TAO)
	Itraconazole (Sporanox)	Voriconazole (Vfend)
	Ketoconazole (Nizoral)	

COMMENTS: Inhibitors of CYP3A4 may increase the serum concentrations of mifepristone. The product information for mifepristone states that strong CYP3A4 inhibitors should be used only with "extreme caution" in patients on mifepristone.

CLASS 2: USE ONLY IF BENEFIT FELT TO OUTWEIGH RISK

• *Use Alternative*:
Azole Antifungals: Fluconazole appears to be a weaker inhibitor of CYP3A4 than itraconazole or ketoconazole. In larger doses it may inhibit CYP3A4 and should be used cautiously with mifepristone. Single doses of fluconazole would be unlikely to increase the risk of mifepristone toxicity. **Terbinafine** (Lamisil) does not appear to inhibit CYP3A4.
Macrolides: Unlike other macrolides, **azithromycin** (Zithromax) and **dirithromycin*** do not appear to inhibit CYP3A4 and would not be expected to interact with mifepristone. (*not available in US)
Telithromycin: The use of **azithromycin** (Zithromax) or a quinolone antibiotic should be considered.

• *Circumvent/Minimize*: In patients receiving strong CYP3A4 inhibitors the product information states that the mifepristone dose should be no higher than 300 mg daily.

• *Monitor*: Monitor for altered mifepristone effect if CYP3A4 inhibitors are initiated, discontinued, or changed in dosage. Adjustments in mifepristone dosage may be necessary.

OBJECT DRUGS	PRECIPITANT DRUGS	
Mifepristone (Korlym)	**Enzyme Inhibitors:**	
	Amiodarone (Cordarone)	Dronedarone (Multaq)
	Amprenavir (Agenerase)	Grapefruit
	Aprepitant (Emend)	Imatinib (Gleevec)
	Atazanavir (Reyataz)	Indinavir (Crixivan)
	Boceprevir (Victrelis)	Lapatinib (Tykerb)
	Ceritinib (Zykadia)	Nelfinavir (Viracept)
	Conivaptan (Vaprisol)	Ritonavir (Norvir)
	Cyclosporine (Neoral)	Saquinavir (Invirase)
	Darunavir (Prezista)	Telaprevir (Incivek)
	Delavirdine (Rescriptor)	Verapamil (Isoptin)
	Diltiazem (Cardizem)	

COMMENTS: Inhibitors of CYP3A4 may increase the serum concentrations of mifepristone. The product information for mifepristone states that strong CYP3A4 inhibitors should be used only with "extreme caution" in patients on mifepristone.

CLASS 2: USE ONLY IF BENEFIT FELT TO OUTWEIGH RISK

• *Use Alternative*:
Calcium channel blockers: Calcium channel blockers other than diltiazem and verapamil are unlikely to inhibit the metabolism of mifepristone.
Grapefruit: Orange juice does not appear to inhibit CYP3A4.

• *Circumvent/Minimize*: In patients receiving strong CYP3A4 inhibitors the product information states that the mifepristone dose should be no higher than 300 mg daily.

• *Monitor*: Monitor for altered mifepristone effect if CYP3A4 inhibitors are initiated, discontinued, or changed in dosage. Adjustments in mifepristone dosage may be necessary.

OBJECT DRUGS	PRECIPITANT DRUGS
Mycophenolate (CellCept)	**Antibiotics:** **Amoxicillin/clavulanate** (Augmentin) **Ciprofloxacin** (Cipro) **Metronidazole** (Flagyl)

COMMENTS: Several studies in transplant patients and healthy subjects have shown that amoxicillin and ciprofloxacin can reduce plasma concentrations of mycophenolic acid (MPA, the active metabolite of mycophenolate). In one case a patient died of severe graft-versus-host disease after ciprofloxacin was added and the AUC of MPA fell to one-third of previous values. Metronidazole has also been reported to reduce MPA concentrations, but the effect may not be as large as with amoxicillin/clavulanate or ciprofloxacin. MPA is excreted in the bile as an inactive glucuronide metabolite, and glucuronidases in intestinal bacteria metabolize the glucuronide back to MPA, which can be reabsorbed. The interaction is thought to result from antibiotic-induced reduction in these bacteria, thus interrupting the enterohepatic recirculation and decreasing MPA plasma concentrations. In one case, intravenous ciprofloxacin appeared to reduce MPA plasma concentrations. Other fluoroquinolones (and perhaps some other antibiotics) may have a similar effect on mycophenolate. Norfloxacin appeared to have an additive effect with metronidazole in reducing MPA concentrations in one study but, norfloxacin given alone had little effect. A small study found reduced MPA concentrations following bowel decontamination with tobramycin plus cefuroxime. Available evidence suggests that co-trimoxazole (trimethoprim/sulfamethoxazole) does not interact with mycophenolate.

CLASS 3: ASSESS RISK & TAKE ACTION IF NECESSARY
- ***Monitor:*** Monitor for altered mycophenolate response if ciprofloxacin, amoxicillin/clavulanate, or other antibiotics are given concurrently. At least some patients may manifest large enough reductions in MPA concentrations to increase the risk of graft-versus-host disease.

OBJECT DRUGS	PRECIPITANT DRUGS
Mycophenolate (CellCept)	**Binding Agents:** **Antacids** **Calcium Polycarbophil** (FiberCon, Konsyl) **Cholestyramine** (Questran) **Colestipol** (Colestid) **Iron** **Sevelamer** (Renagel) **Sucralfate** (Carafate)

COMMENTS: Cholestyramine can substantially reduce mycophenolate mofetil (MM) serum concentrations by binding in the gastrointestinal tract and interfering with its enterohepatic circulation. Colestipol theoretically would have a similar effect. Aluminum-magnesium antacids modestly reduce MM absorption. The effect of iron on MM may be less in patients taking cyclosporine plus MM.

CLASS 3: ASSESS RISK & TAKE ACTION IF NECESSARY
- ***Circumvent/Minimize:*** Since the interaction appears to be due to interruption of MM enterohepatic circulation, separation of doses is not likely to circumvent the interaction completely. Nonetheless, if the combination is used, separate the doses as much as possible and monitor for reduced MM effect.
- ***Consider Alternative:***
  Lipid Lowering Agents: The use of alternative hypolipidemic such as HMG-CoA reductase inhibitors should be considered. The effect of **colesevelam** (Welchol) on MM is not established, but it might interact.
  Antacids: Antisecretory agents such as H_2-receptor antagonists or proton pump inhibitors would be less likely to interact than antacids.
- ***Monitor:*** Patients receiving mycophenolate with binding resins or antacids should be monitored for reduced immunosuppressant efficacy.

OBJECT DRUGS	PRECIPITANT DRUGS	
Mycophenolate (CellCept)	**Gastric Antisecretory Agents:**	
	Cimetidine (Tagamet)	**Nizatidine** (Axid)
	Dexlansoprazole (Kapidex)	**Omeprazole** (Prilosec)
	Esomeprazole (Nexium)	**Pantoprazole** (Protonix)
	Famotidine (Pepcid)	**Rabeprazole** (Aciphex)
	Lansoprazole (Prevacid)	**Ranitidine** (Zantac)

COMMENTS: Mycophenolate dissolution is reduced by agents that increase gastric pH resulting in a reduction of mycophenolate absorption and plasma concentration of mycophenolate.

CLASS 3: ASSESS RISK & TAKE ACTION IF NECESSARY
- *Consider Alternative*: Enteric coated mycophenolate acid is not affected by changes in gastric acidity.
- *Monitor*: Monitor for altered immunosuppressive response if a gastric antisecretory agent is initiated, discontinued, or changed in dosage.

OBJECT DRUGS	PRECIPITANT DRUGS
Nitrates:	**Vasodilators:**
Isosorbide Dinitrate (Isordil)	**Avanafil** (Stendra)
Isosorbide Mononitrate (Ismo)	**Riociguat** (Adempas)
Nitroglycerin (Nitrogard)	**Sildenafil** (Viagra)
	Tadalafil (Cialis)
	Vardenafil (Levitra)

COMMENTS: Vasodilators may markedly enhance the hypotensive effects of nitrates. Fatalities have been reported, although a causal relationship was not established in some cases. Other vasodilators such as **terazosin** (Hytrin) and **doxazosin** (Cardura) have also been reported to produce hypotensive episodes when coadministered with these drugs.

CLASS 1: AVOID COMBINATION
- *Avoid*: Patients taking nitrates by any route of administration should avoid taking these vasodilators.

OBJECT DRUGS		PRECIPITANT DRUGS
NSAIDs:		**SSRI and SNRI:**
Diclofenac (Voltaren)	**Meclofenamate**	**Citalopram** (Celexa)
Diflunisal (Dolobid)	**Mefenamic acid**	**Clomipramine** (Anafranil)
Etodolac (Lodine)	**Meloxicam** (Mobic)	**Desvenlafaxine** (Pristiq)
Fenoprofen (Nalfon)	**Nabumetone** (Relafen)	**Duloxetine** (Cymbalta)
Flurbiprofen (Ansaid)	**Naproxen** (Aleve)	**Escitalopram** (Lexapro)
Ibuprofen (Motrin)	**Oxaprozin** (Daypro)	**Fluoxetine** (Prozac)
Indomethacin (Indocin)	**Piroxicam** (Feldene)	**Fluvoxamine** (Luvox)
Ketoprofen (Orudis)	**Sulindac** (Clinoril)	**Imipramine** (Tofranil)
Ketorolac (Toradol)	**Tolmetin** (Tolectin)	**Levomilnacipran** (Fetzima)
		Milnacipran (Savella)
		Nefazodone
		Paroxetine (Paxil)
		Sertraline (Zoloft)
		Venlafaxine (Effexor)
		Vilazodone (Viibryd)
		Vortioxetine (Brintellix)

COMMENTS: Some studies suggest that the concurrent use of NSAIDs or aspirin with serotonin reuptake inhibitors (SSRI) or serotonin-norepinephrine uptake inhibitors (SNRI) increases the risk of gastrointestinal (GI) bleeding compared to either drug used alone. Some evidence suggests that even low-dose aspirin may increase GI bleeding when combined with SSRIs or SNRIs. However, the vast majority of patients on concurrent therapy with an NSAID or aspirin and an SSRI will not develop GI bleeding. Since GI bleeding can be fatal, however, anything that increases the risk should be avoided if possible. The putative mechanism is inhibition of serotonin uptake by platelets added to gastric toxicity and antiplatelet effect caused by the NSAIDs. The risk of GI bleeding appears to be related to the potency of the serotonin reuptake inhibition, a finding that lends additional support to the existence of an interaction.

CLASS 3: ASSESS RISK & TAKE ACTION IF NECESSARY
- *Consider Alternative*:
  NSAIDs: If the NSAID is being used as an analgesic, consider using acetaminophen instead. COX-2 inhibitors do not affect platelets, and may offer a lower risk of GI bleeding when combined with a SSRI.
  Antidepressant: If appropriate for the patient, consider using agents with low serotonin reuptake inhibition such as **desipramine** (Norpramin), **maprotiline** (Ludiomil), **nortriptyline** (Aventyl), **trimipramine** (Surmontil) or moderate serotonin reuptake inhibitors such as **amitriptyline** (Elavil) or **imipramine** (Tofranil).
- *Monitor*: Patients and health professionals should be alert for evidence of gastrointestinal bleeding if these combinations are used.

OBJECT DRUGS	PRECIPITANT DRUGS	
Opioid Analgesics:	**Enzyme Inducers:**	
Alfentanil (Alfenta)	**Barbiturates**	**Oxcarbazepine** (Trileptal)
Codeine	**Bosentan** (Tracleer)	**Phenytoin** (Dilantin)
Fentanyl (Sublimaze)	**Carbamazepine** (Tegretol)	**Primidone** (Mysoline)
Methadone (Dolophine)	**Dabrafenib** (Tafinlar)	**Rifampin** (Rifadin)
Morphine	**Efavirenz** (Sustiva)	**Rifapentine** (Priftin)
Oxycodone (Percocet)	**Etravirine** (Intelence)	**Ritonavir** (Norvir)
Sufentanil (Sufenta)	**Lumacaftor** (Orkambi)	**St. John's wort**
	Nevirapine (Viramune)	

COMMENTS: Enzyme inducers may increase the elimination of these opioids via CYP3A4 metabolism and possibly other pathways. This may result in reduced analgesic effects and may cause withdrawal symptoms in patients maintained on methadone. For example, rifampin has been shown to markedly reduce oxycodone plasma concentrations. Potent enzyme inducers such as rifampin may have larger effects on these analgesics than other inducers. With codeine, rifampin reduced the conversion of codeine to morphine, but only in those with normal CYP2D6 activity (EMs). Rifampin did not interact with codeine in subjects with little CYP2D6 activity (PMs), but PMs are not likely to have adequate analgesic effects from codeine whether or not they are taking enzyme inducers such as rifampin. Ritonavir may have variable effects on these opioids, depending on the duration of ritonavir therapy and other factors. In one study, ritonavir *increased* fentanyl plasma concentrations.

CLASS 3: ASSESS RISK & TAKE ACTION IF NECESSARY
- *Consider Alternative*: While it would be prudent to use an alternative to the enzyme inducer, suitable alternatives with equivalent therapeutic effects are not available for most enzyme inducers.
- *Monitor*: Monitor for reduced analgesic effect or evidence of methadone withdrawal (e.g., rhinorrhea, sweating, lacrimation, restlessness, and insomnia). Increase dose of opioid if needed. If the dose of the opioid is increased to compensate for the enzyme inducer, monitor for opioid toxicity if the enzyme inducer is stopped or reduced in dosage. Keep in mind that enzyme induction is usually gradual and may take days to weeks for onset and offset, depending on the specific inducer.

OBJECT DRUGS	PRECIPITANT DRUGS	
Opioid Analgesics:	**Antimicrobials:**	
Alfentanil (Alfenta)	**Ciprofloxacin** (Cipro)	**Ketoconazole** (Nizoral)
Fentanyl (Sublimaze)	**Clarithromycin** (Biaxin)	**Posaconazole** (Noxafil)
Methadone (Dolophine)	**Clotrimazole** (Mycelex)	**Quinupristin** (Synercid)
Oxycodone (Percocet)	**Erythromycin** (E-Mycin)	**Telithromycin** (Ketek)
Sufentanil (Sufenta)	**Fluconazole** (Diflucan)	**Troleandomycin** (TAO)
	Itraconazole (Sporanox)	**Voriconazole** (Vfend)

COMMENTS: These antimicrobials inhibit CYP3A4 and may inhibit the elimination of these opioids via CYP3A4 metabolism and possibly other pathways. Excessive opioid effects have been reported. For example, voriconazole produced almost a 4-fold increase in oxycodone plasma concentrations.

CLASS 3: ASSESS RISK & TAKE ACTION IF NECESSARY
- *Consider Alternative*:
  Azole Antifungals: Itraconazole and ketoconazole are potent inhibitors of CYP3A4; fluconazole appears weaker, but in larger doses it also inhibits CYP3A4. **Terbinafine** (Lamisil) does not appear to affect CYP3A4.

Macrolide Antibiotics: Unlike erythromycin, clarithromycin and troleandomycin, **azithromycin** (Zithromax) and **dirithromycin*** do not appear to inhibit CYP3A4. (*not available in US) Telithromycin: The use of **azithromycin** (Zithromax) or a quinolone antibiotic other than ciprofloxacin should be considered.
- *Monitor*: Monitor for evidence of excessive and/or prolonged opioid effects, including sedation and respiratory depression.

OBJECT DRUGS	PRECIPITANT DRUGS	
Opioid Analgesics:	**Enzyme Inhibitors:**	
Alfentanil (Alfenta)	**Amiodarone** Cordarone)	**Dronedarone** (Multaq)
Fentanyl (Sublimaze)	**Amprenavir** (Agenerase)	**Fluvoxamine** (Luvox)
Methadone (Dolophine)	**Aprepitant** (Emend)	**Grapefruit**
Oxycodone (Percocet)	**Atazanavir** (Reyataz)	**Indinavir** (Crixivan)
Sufentanil (Sufenta)	**Boceprevir** (Victrelis)	**Lomitapide** (Juxtapid)
	Ceritinib (Zykadia)	**Mifepristone** (Korlym)
	Cimetidine (Tagamet)	**Nefazodone**
	Cobicistat (Stribild)	**Nelfinavir** (Viracept)
	Conivaptan (Vaprisol)	**Ritonavir** (Norvir)
	Cyclosporine (Neoral)	**Saquinavir** (Invirase)
	Darunavir (Prezista)	**Telaprevir** (Incivek)
	Delavirdine (Rescriptor)	**Verapamil** (Isoptin)
	Diltiazem (Cardizem)	

COMMENTS: These enzyme inhibitors may inhibit the elimination of these opioids via CYP3A4 metabolism and possibly other pathways. Excessive opioid effects have been reported. The magnitude of the interaction may vary considerably depending on the inhibitor. Some inhibitors (e.g., cyclosporine, nefazodone) are more potent than weaker inhibitors such as cimetidine. Nonetheless, cimetidine produced a large increase in alfentanil half-life and large reduction in alfentanil clearance (ranitidine had no effect). In patients on methadone maintenance amprenavir modestly *decreased* R- and S- methadone plasma concentrations, suggesting that amprenavir can act as both an inhibitor and an inducer of CYP3A4. There was no evidence of methadone withdrawal in the patients, but patients on the combination should be monitored for altered methadone response. The mifepristone product information states that concurrent use of fentanyl is contraindicated.

CLASS 3: ASSESS RISK & TAKE ACTION IF NECESSARY
- *Consider Alternative*:
Calcium channel blockers: Calcium channel blockers other than diltiazem and verapamil are unlikely to inhibit CYP3A4.
Cimetidine: **Famotidine** (Pepcid), **nizatidine** (Axid), and **ranitidine** (Zantac) have minimal effects on drug metabolism.
Grapefruit: Orange juice does not appear to inhibit CYP3A4.
Antidepressants: **Sertraline** (Zoloft), **citalopram** (Celexa), **venlafaxine** (Effexor), and **paroxetine** (Paxil) appear less likely to inhibit CYP3A4 than fluvoxamine, and much less likely than nefazodone. **Fluoxetine** (Prozac) appears to be a weak inhibitor of CYP3A4.
- *Monitor*: Monitor for evidence of excessive and/or prolonged opioid effects, including sedation and respiratory depression.

OBJECT DRUGS	PRECIPITANT DRUGS	
Opioid Analgesics	SSRI and SNRI:	Levomilnacipran (Fetzima)
(Serotonergic):	Citalopram (Celexa)	Imipramine (Tofranil)
Alfentanil (Alfenta)	Clomipramine (Anafranil)	Milnacipran (Savella)
Fentanyl (Sublimaze)	Desvenlafaxine (Pristiq)	Paroxetine (Paxil)
Meperidine (Demerol)	Duloxetine (Cymbalta)	Sertraline (Zoloft)
Methadone (Dolophine)	Escitalopram (Lexapro)	Venlafaxine (Effexor)
Tapentadol (Nucynta)	Fluoxetine (Prozac)	Vilazodone (Viibryd)
Tramadol (Ultram)	Fluvoxamine (Luvox)	Vortioxetine (Brintellix)

COMMENTS: There have been a number of cases of serotonin syndrome following the combined use of serotonergic analgesics such as meperidine or tramadol with selective serotonin reuptake inhibitors (SSRI) or selective serotonin-norepinephrine reuptake inhibitors (SNRI). One case of fatal serotonin syndrome was reported in a patient on **amitriptyline** following the addition of tramadol. Limited evidence suggests that **fentanyl** may also exhibit additive serotonergic effects with other serotonergic drugs, but more evidence is needed. Use particular care if the SSRI or SNRI is also an inhibitor of the metabolism of the opioid.

CLASS 3: ASSESS RISK & TAKE ACTION IF NECESSARY

- *Consider Alternative*:
  Opioid Analgesic: In patients taking an SSRI or SNRI consider using an alternative to the serotonergic opioid.
  Antidepressant: If a tricyclic antidepressant (TCA) is given to patients on a serotonergic opioid, use a TCA other than clomipramine or imipramine. Avoiding **amitriptyline, doxepin** and **desipramine** would also be prudent.
- *Monitor:* Monitor for evidence of serotonin toxicity (myoclonus, rigidity, tremor, fever, sweating, seizures, confusion, agitation, incoordination, and coma).

OBJECT DRUGS	PRECIPITANT DRUGS	
Phenytoin (Dilantin)	Enzyme Inhibitors:	
	Amiodarone (Cordarone)	Fluorouracil (5-FU)
	Androgens	Fluoxetine (Prozac)
	Capecitabine (Xeloda)	Fluvoxamine (Luvox)
	Ceritinib (Zykadia)	Imatinib (Gleevec)
	Chloramphenicol	Isoniazid (INH)
	Cimetidine (Tagamet)	Leflunomide (Arava)
	Co-trimoxazole (Bactrim)	Metronidazole (Flagyl)
	Danazol (Danocrine)	Sulfinpyrazone (Anturane)
	Delavirdine (Rescriptor)	Tamoxifen (Nolvadex)
	Disulfiram (Antabuse)	Ticlopidine (Ticlid)
	Efavirenz (Sustiva)	Voriconazole (Vfend)
	Fluconazole (Diflucan)	

COMMENTS: Inhibitors of CYP2C9 (and to a lesser extent CYP2C19) may increase phenytoin and **fosphenytoin** (Cerebyx) levels; phenytoin toxicity may occur. Depending on the baseline phenytoin serum concentration, it may take as long as several weeks for phenytoin toxicity to occur after starting an inhibitor. If isoniazid is combined with rifampin in a patient on phenytoin, phenytoin concentrations may actually *decrease* because the enzyme induction produced by rifampin may outweigh the enzyme inhibition of the isoniazid. Also, keep in mind that phenytoin induces several CYP450 isozymes (CYP3A4, CYP2C9, CYP1A2, etc.) and it may reduce the plasma concentrations of many of the inhibitors listed here.

CLASS 3: ASSESS RISK & TAKE ACTION IF NECESSARY

- *Consider Alternative*:
  Azole Antifungals: Ketoconazole (Nizoral), **posaconazole** (Noxafil), and **itraconazole** (Sporanox) appear to be less likely to affect phenytoin.
  Cimetidine: **Famotidine** (Pepcid), **nizatidine** (Axid), and **ranitidine** (Zantac) have minimal effects on drug metabolism.
  Fluvastatin: Statins other than fluvastatin do not appear to inhibit CYP2C9.
  SSRIs: The use of SSRIs that do not inhibit CYP2C9 [eg, **paroxetine** (Paxil) or **venlafaxine** (Effexor)] should be considered.
- *Monitor:* Monitor for altered phenytoin effect if an inhibitor is initiated, discontinued, or changed in dosage. Evidence of phenytoin toxicity includes nystagmus, ataxia, diplopia, drowsiness, and lethargy; severe cases may result in asterixis and coma.

OBJECT DRUGS	PRECIPITANT DRUGS
Phosphodiesterase Inhibitors: **Avanafil** (Stendra) **Sildenafil** (Viagra) **Tadalafil** (Cialis) **Vardenafil** (Levitra)	**Antidepressants:** **Fluvoxamine** (Luvox) **Nefazodone**

COMMENTS: The phosphodiesterase inhibitors are metabolized by CYP3A4 and concurrent administration with CYP3A4 inhibitors could produce increased plasma concentrations. Increased side effects may occur during coadministered with CYP3A4 inhibitors.

CLASS 3: ASSESS RISK & TAKE ACTION IF NECESSARY
- *Consider Alternative*: Sertraline (Zoloft), **venlafaxine** (Effexor), **paroxetine** (Paxil), **citalopram** (Celexa), and **escitalopram** (Lexapro) are not known to inhibit CYP3A4. **Fluoxetine** (Prozac) appears to be a weak CYP3A4 inhibitor.
- *Monitor*: Monitor for phosphodiesterase inhibitor toxicity including visual disturbances, hypotension, and syncope. Reduced dose of the phosphodiesterase inhibitor may be required.

OBJECT DRUGS	PRECIPITANT DRUGS	
Phosphodiesterase Inhibitors: **Avanafil** (Stendra) **Sildenafil** (Viagra) **Tadalafil** (Cialis) **Vardenafil** (Levitra)	**Antimicrobials:** **Ciprofloxacin** (Cipro) **Clarithromycin** (Biaxin) **Erythromycin** (E-Mycin) **Fluconazole** (Diflucan) **Itraconazole** (Sporanox) **Ketoconazole** (Nizoral)	**Posaconazole** (Noxafil) **Quinupristin** (Synercid) **Telithromycin** (Ketek) **Troleandomycin** (TAO) **Voriconazole** (Vfend)

COMMENTS: The phosphodiesterase inhibitors appear to be metabolized by CYP3A4 and concurrent administration with CYP3A4 inhibitors could produce increased plasma concentrations. Increased side effects may occur with concurrent CYP3A4 inhibitors.

CLASS 3: ASSESS RISK & TAKE ACTION IF NECESSARY
- *Consider Alternative*:
- Azole Antifungals: Itraconazole and ketoconazole are potent inhibitors of CYP3A4; fluconazole appears weaker, but in larger doses it also inhibits CYP3A4. **Terbinafine** (Lamisil) does not appear to affect CYP3A4, and would not be expected to interact with phosphodiesterase inhibitors.
  Macrolide Antibiotics: Unlike erythromycin, clarithromycin and troleandomycin, **azithromycin** (Zithromax) and **dirithromycin*** do not appear to inhibit CYP3A4. (*not available in US*)
  Telithromycin: The use of **azithromycin** (Zithromax) or a quinolone antibiotic other than ciprofloxacin should be considered.
- *Monitor*: Monitor for phosphodiesterase inhibitor toxicity including visual disturbances, hypotension, and syncope. Reduced dose of the phosphodiesterase inhibitor may be required.

OBJECT DRUGS	PRECIPITANT DRUGS
Phosphodiesterase Inhibitors: **Avanafil** (Stendra) **Sildenafil** (Viagra) **Tadalafil** (Cialis) **Vardenafil** (Levitra)	**Calcium Channel Blockers:** **Diltiazem** (Cardizem) **Verapamil** (Isoptin)

COMMENTS: The phosphodiesterase inhibitors appear to be metabolized by CYP3A4 and concurrent administration with CYP3A4 inhibitors such as diltiazem and verapamil could produce increased plasma concentrations. Increased side effects may occur during coadministered with CYP3A4 inhibitors.

CLASS 3: ASSESS RISK & TAKE ACTION IF NECESSARY
- *Consider Alternative*: Calcium channel blockers other than diltiazem and verapamil are unlikely to inhibit the metabolism of sildenafil. However, other calcium channel blockers may produce increased hypotensive effects when used with phosphodiesterase inhibitors.
- *Monitor*: Monitor for phosphodiesterase inhibitor toxicity including visual disturbances, hypotension, and syncope. Reduced dose of the phosphodiesterase inhibitor may be required.

OBJECT DRUGS	PRECIPITANT DRUGS	
Phosphodiesterase Inhibitors:	**Enzyme Inhibitors:**	
Avanafil (Stendra)	**Amiodarone** (Cordarone)	**Delavirdine** (Rescriptor)
Sildenafil (Viagra)	**Amprenavir** (Agenerase)	**Dronedarone** (Multaq)
Tadalafil (Cialis)	**Aprepitant** (Emend)	**Grapefruit**
Vardenafil (Levitra)	**Atazanavir** (Reyataz)	**Indinavir** (Crixivan)
	Boceprevir (Victrelis)	**Lomitapide** (Juxtapid)
	Ceritinib (Zykadia)	**Mifepristone** (Korlym)
	Cobicistat (Stribild)	**Nelfinavir** (Viracept)
	Cimetidine (Tagamet)	**Ritonavir** (Norvir)
	Conivaptan (Vaprisol)	**Saquinavir** (Invirase)
	Cyclosporine (Neoral)	**Telaprevir** (Incivek)
	Darunavir (Prezista)	

COMMENTS: The phosphodiesterase inhibitors are metabolized by CYP3A4; concurrent administration with CYP3A4 inhibitors could produce increased plasma concentrations. Increased side effects may occur during coadministration with CYP3A4 inhibitors.

CLASS 3: ASSESS RISK & TAKE ACTION IF NECESSARY
- *Consider Alternative*:
  Cimetidine: **Famotidine** (Pepcid), **nizatidine** (Axid), and **ranitidine** (Zantac) have minimal effects on drug metabolism.
  Grapefruit: Orange juice does not appear to inhibit CYP3A4.
- *Monitor:* Monitor for phosphodiesterase inhibitor toxicity including visual disturbances, hypotension, and syncope. Reduced dose of the phosphodiesterase inhibitor may be required.

OBJECT DRUGS	PRECIPITANT DRUGS	
Pimozide (Orap)	**Antimicrobials:**	
	Ciprofloxacin (Cipro)	**Posaconazole** (Noxafil)
	Clarithromycin (Biaxin)	**Quinupristin** (Synercid)
	Erythromycin (E-Mycin)	**Telithromycin** (Ketek)
	Fluconazole (Diflucan)	**Troleandomycin** (TAO)
	Itraconazole (Sporanox)	**Voriconazole** (Vfend)
	Ketoconazole (Nizoral)	

COMMENTS: Pimozide alone can prolong the QT interval, and it has been associated with ventricular arrhythmias (torsades de pointes). Drugs that inhibit CYP3A4 may increase pimozide serum concentrations.

CLASS 1: AVOID COMBINATION
- *Avoid:* These antimicrobials should not be given to patients receiving pimozide due to the risk of life-threatening ventricular arrhythmias.
- *Use Alternative*:
  Azole Antifungals: Itraconazole and ketoconazole are potent inhibitors of CYP3A4: fluconazole appears weaker, but in larger doses it also inhibits CYP3A4. **Terbinafine** (Lamisil) does not appear to affect CYP3A4, and would not be expected to interact with pimozide.
  Macrolide Antibiotics: Unlike erythromycin, clarithromycin and troleandomycin, **azithromycin** (Zithromax) and **dirithromycin*** do not appear to inhibit CYP3A4. (*not available in US)
  Telithromycin: The use of **azithromycin** (Zithromax) or a quinolone antibiotic other than ciprofloxacin could be considered.

OBJECT DRUGS	PRECIPITANT DRUGS	
Pimozide (Orap)	**Enzyme Inhibitors:**	
	Amiodarone (Cordarone)	**Dronedarone** (Multaq)
	Amprenavir (Agenerase)	**Fluvoxamine** (Luvox)
	Aprepitant (Emend)	**Grapefruit**
	Atazanavir (Reyataz)	**Indinavir** (Crixivan)
	Boceprevir (Victrelis)	**Lomitapide** (Juxtapid)
	Ceritinib (Zykadia)	**Mifepristone** (Korlym)
	Cobicistat (Stribild)	**Nefazodone**
	Conivaptan (Vaprisol)	**Nelfinavir** (Viracept)
	Cyclosporine (Neoral)	**Ritonavir** (Norvir)
	Darunavir (Prezista)	**Saquinavir** (Invirase)
	Delavirdine (Rescriptor)	**Telaprevir** (Incivek)
	Diltiazem (Cardizem)	**Verapamil** (Isoptin)

COMMENTS: Pimozide alone can prolong the QT interval, and it has been associated with ventricular arrhythmias (torsades de pointes). Drugs that inhibit CYP3A4 may increase pimozide serum concentrations and increase the risk of ventricular arrhythmias. Orap product information states that pimozide is contraindicated with indinavir, nelfinavir, ritonavir, saquinavir, and other CYP3A4 inhibitors. The mifepristone product information states that concurrent use of pimozide is contraindicated.

CLASS 1: AVOID COMBINATION
• *Avoid:* CYP3A4 inhibitors should not be given to patients receiving pimozide due to the risk of life-threatening ventricular arrhythmias. Use an alternative drug to the CYP3A4 inhibitor if possible.
• *Use Alternative:*
Antidepressants: Citalopram (Celexa), venlafaxine (Effexor), and paroxetine (Paxil) appear less likely to inhibit CYP3A4 than fluvoxamine. Fluoxetine (Prozac) appears to be a weak inhibitor of CYP3A4, and could increase pimozide concentrations.
Calcium channel blockers: Calcium channel blockers other than diltiazem and verapamil are unlikely to inhibit CYP3A4.
Grapefruit: Orange juice does not appear to inhibit CYP3A4.

OBJECT DRUGS	PRECIPITANT DRUGS	
Potassium-sparing diuretics:	**ACE inhibitors:**	
Amiloride (Midamor)	**Benazepril** (Lotensin)	**Moexipril** (Univasc)
Eplerenone (Inspra)	**Captopril** (Capoten)	**Perindopril** (Aceon)
Spironolactone (Aldactone)	**Enalapril** (Vasotec)	**Quinapril** (Accupril)
Triamterene (Dyrenium)	**Fosinopril** (Monopril)	**Ramipril** (Altace)
	Lisinopril (Prinivil)	**Trandolapril** (Mavik)

COMMENTS: Concurrent use of potassium sparing diuretics and ACE inhibitors may lead to additive hyperkalemic effects and excessive serum potassium levels, especially in the presence of one or more predisposing factors such as significant renal impairment, severe diabetes, potassium supplements, high potassium diet, and advanced age. Fatal hyperkalemia has occurred, but is probably rare. ACE inhibitors are frequently used with potassium-sparing diuretics with good results, but close monitoring is necessary in patients with risk factors. Other drugs that may exhibit hyperkalemic activity include **drospirenone** (Yasmin), **heparins, nonselective beta-blockers, NSAIDs, COX-2 inhibitors, angiotensin receptor blockers, cyclosporine, tacrolimus, succinylcholine, pentamidine, trimethoprim,** and **potassium-containing salt substitutes.**

CLASS 3: ASSESS RISK & TAKE ACTION IF NECESSARY
• *Monitor:* Monitor serum potassium concentrations, especially in patients with predisposing factors such as renal disease, diabetes, and advanced age.

OBJECT DRUGS	PRECIPITANT DRUGS
Potassium-sparing diuretics:	**Angiotensin Receptor Blockers:**
Amiloride (Midamor)	**Azilsartan** (Edarbi)
Eplerenone (Inspra)	**Candesartan** (Atacand)
Spironolactone (Aldactone)	**Eprosartan** (Teveten)
Triamterene (Dyrenium)	**Irbesartan** (Avapro)
	Losartan (Cozaar)
	Olmesartan (Benicar)
	Telmisartan (Micardis)
	Valsartan (Diovan)

COMMENTS: Concurrent use of potassium-sparing diuretics and angiotensin receptor blockers (ARBs) may lead to additive hyperkalemic effects and excessive serum potassium levels, especially in the presence of one or more predisposing factors such as significant renal impairment, severe diabetes, potassium supplements, high potassium diet, and advanced age. Fatal hyperkalemia has occurred, but is rare. ARBs are frequently used with potassium-sparing diuretics with good results, but close monitoring is necessary in patients with risk factors. Other drugs that may exhibit hyperkalemic activity include **ACE inhibitors, drospirenone** (Yasmin), **heparins, nonselective beta-blockers, NSAIDs, COX-2 inhibitors, cyclosporine, tacrolimus, succinylcholine, pentamidine, trimethoprim,** and **potassium-containing salt substitutes.**

CLASS 3: ASSESS RISK & TAKE ACTION IF NECESSARY
- *Monitor:* Monitor serum potassium concentrations, especially in patients with predisposing factors such as renal disease, diabetes, and advanced age.

OBJECT DRUGS	PRECIPITANT DRUGS
Procainamide (Pronestyl)	**Cimetidine** (Tagamet)
	Co-trimoxazole (Bactrim, Septra)
	Ketoconazole (Nizoral)
	Levofloxacin (Levaquin)
	Triamterene (Dyrenium)

COMMENTS: The renal clearance of procainamide may be reduced by these drugs, resulting in elevated procainamide concentrations, particularly in patients with renal dysfunction. Pending more study, other drugs reported to inhibit cationic tubular secretion (e.g., **amiodarone, dofetilide, diltiazem, metformin,** and **verapamil**) should be used with careful monitoring in patients taking procainamide.

CLASS 3: ASSESS RISK & TAKE ACTION IF NECESSARY
- *Consider Alternative:*
  Cimetidine: Other H$_2$-receptor antagonists such as **famotidine** (Pepcid), **nizatidine** (Axid), and **ranitidine** (Zantac) could be used instead of cimetidine.
  Triamterene: **Spironolactone** (Aldactone) or **amiloride** (Midamor) could be used as a potassium-sparing diuretic.
- *Monitor:* Be alert for increased procainamide effects (e.g., prolonged QRS or QTc intervals) in patients taking drugs that are known to reduce cationic renal clearance.

OBJECT DRUGS	PRECIPITANT DRUGS
Quinolones:	**Binding Agents:**
Ciprofloxacin (Cipro)	**Antacids**
Enoxacin (Penetrex)	**Calcium Polycarbophil** (FiberCon)
Gemifloxacin (Factive)	**Didanosine** (Videx)
Levofloxacin (Levaquin)	**Iron**
Lomefloxacin (Maxaquin)	**Sucralfate** (Carafate)
Moxifloxacin (Avelox)	**Zinc**
Norfloxacin (Noroxin)	
Ofloxacin (Floxin)	
Sparfloxacin (Zagam)	

COMMENTS: The absorption of quinolones is markedly reduced by agents containing cations such as aluminum, magnesium, and to a lesser extent, iron and calcium. Ciprofloxacin and norfloxacin appear more susceptible to this effect than lomefloxacin or ofloxacin; iron has little effect on lomefloxacin and ofloxacin. Limited evidence suggests that the absorption of some quinolones may be affected by multivitamins with minerals.

CLASS 3: ASSESS RISK & TAKE ACTION IF NECESSARY
* *Consider Alternative:* Calcium carbonate does not impair quinolone absorption as much as aluminum-magnesium antacids, but it would still be prudent to separate doses. Gatifloxacin absorption does not appear to be affected by calcium carbonate. Enteric coated didanosine (Videx EC) does not interact.
* *Circumvent/Minimize:* Giving the quinolone 2 hours before or 6 hours after the cation minimizes the interaction.
* *Monitor:* Watch for reduced quinolone antibiotic efficacy in patients taking di- or trivalent cations.

OBJECT DRUGS	PRECIPITANT DRUGS
Ramelteon (Rozerem)	**Enzyme Inhibitors:**
Tasimelteon (Hetlioz)	**Atazanavir** (Reyataz)
	Cimetidine (Tagamet)
	Ciprofloxacin (Cipro)
	Enoxacin (Penetrex)
	Fluvoxamine (Luvox)
	Mexiletine (Mexitil)
	Tacrine (Cognex)
	Zileuton (Zyflo)

COMMENTS: Ramelteon is metabolized by CYP1A2, and inhibitors of CYP1A2 can produce dramatic increases in ramelteon plasma concentrations. Fluvoxamine is one of the post potent CYP1A2 inhibitors known, and it can cause an almost 200-fold increase in ramelteon plasma concentrations. Given the apparently high sensitivity of ramelteon to CYP1A2 inhibitors, even weaker inhibitors may be expected to produce substantial increases in ramelteon plasma concentrations. Although ramelteon does not appear to have much dose-related toxicity in normal dose ranges, it is possible that toxicity may occur following the dramatically increased concentrations found after concurrent use of CYP1A2 inhibitors. Tasimelteon is also metabolized by CYP1A2, but is not as sensitive to CYP1A2 inhibitors as ramelteon.

CLASS 2: USE ONLY IF BENEFIT FELT TO OUTWEIGH RISK
* *Use Alternative:* Given the magnitude of the increases in ramelteon plasma concentrations, it would be prudent to avoid these combinations.
  Ramelteon or Tasimelteon: **Eszopiclone** (Lunesta), **zaleplon** (Sonata), **zolpidem** (Ambien), and **zopiclone** (Imovane) are metabolized primarily by CYP3A4, and are probably less likely to interact with CYP1A2 inhibitors than is ramelteon.
  Cimetidine: **Famotidine** (Pepcid), **nizatidine** (Axid), and **ranitidine** (Zantac) do not appear to affect CYP1A2 activity.
  Fluoroquinolones: **Gemifloxacin** (Factive), **levofloxacin** (Levaquin), **lomefloxacin** (Maxaquin), **moxifloxacin** (Avelox), **norfloxacin** (Noroxin), and **ofloxacin** (Floxin) appear to have little effect on CYP1A2.
  Fluvoxamine: **Citalopram** (Celexa), **escitalopram** (Lexapro), **fluoxetine** (Prozac), **paroxetine** (Paxil), **sertraline** (Zoloft), and **venlafaxine** (Effexor), are not known to inhibit CYP1A2.
* *Monitor:* If ramelteon or tasimelteon is used with a CYP1A2 inhibitor, monitor for evidence of ramelteon toxicity.

OBJECT DRUGS	PRECIPITANT DRUGS
Ranolazine (Ranexa)	**Antimicrobials:**

Ciprofloxacin (Cipro)	**Posaconazole** (Noxafil)
Clarithromycin (Biaxin)	**Quinupristin** (Synercid)
Erythromycin (E-Mycin)	**Telithromycin** (Ketek)
Fluconazole (Diflucan)	**Troleandomycin** (TAO)
Itraconazole (Sporanox)	**Voriconazole** (Vfend)
Ketoconazole (Nizoral)	

COMMENTS: Ranolazine is metabolized primarily by CYP3A4, and inhibitors of this isozyme increase the serum concentrations of ranolazine. The product information states that ranolazine is contraindicated with potent or moderately potent CYP3A4 inhibitors. Theoretically, such drugs could increase the risk of ranolazine-induced QTc prolongation and ventricular arrhythmias.

CLASS 2: USE ONLY IF BENEFIT FELT TO OUTWEIGH RISK
- *Use Alternative*:
  Azole Antifungals: Itraconazole and ketoconazole are potent inhibitors of CYP3A4; fluconazole appears weaker, but in larger doses it also inhibits CYP3A4.
  Macrolide Antibiotics: Unlike erythromycin, clarithromycin and troleandomycin, **azithromycin** (Zithromax) and **dirithromycin*** do not appear to inhibit CYP3A4. (*not available in US)
  Telithromycin: The use of **azithromycin** (Zithromax) or a quinolone antibiotic other than ciprofloxacin could be considered.
- *Circumvent/Minimize*: Consider reducing the dose of ranolazine if enzyme inhibitors are coadministered.
- *Monitor*: If the combination is used, the primary concern is QTc prolongation. Monitor the ECG and advise the patient to report any episodes of dizziness or syncope.

OBJECT DRUGS	PRECIPITANT DRUGS
Ranolazine (Ranexa)	**Antidepressants:** **Fluvoxamine** (Luvox) Nefazodone

COMMENTS: Ranolazine is metabolized primarily by CYP3A4, and inhibitors of this isozyme increase the serum concentrations of ranolazine. The product information states that ranolazine is contraindicated with potent (nefazodone) or moderately potent (fluvoxamine) CYP3A4 inhibitors. Theoretically, such drugs could increase the risk of ranolazine-induced QTc prolongation and ventricular arrhythmias.

CLASS 2: USE ONLY IF BENEFIT FELT TO OUTWEIGH RISK
- *Use Alternative*: Sertraline (Zoloft), **citalopram** (Celexa), **escitalopram** (Lexapro), and **venlafaxine** (Effexor), have little effect on CYP3A4.
- *Circumvent/Minimize*: Consider reducing the dose of ranolazine if enzyme inhibitors are coadministered.
- *Monitor*: If the combination is used, the primary concern is QTc prolongation. Monitor the ECG and advise the patient to report any episodes of dizziness or syncope.

OBJECT DRUGS	PRECIPITANT DRUGS	
Ranolazine (Ranexa)	**Enzyme Inhibitors:**	
	Amiodarone (Cordarone)	**Diltiazem** (Cardizem)
	Amprenavir (Agenerase)	**Dronedarone** (Multaq)
	Aprepitant (Emend)	**Grapefruit**
	Atazanavir (Reyataz)	**Indinavir** (Crixivan)
	Boceprevir (Victrelis)	**Lomitapide** (Juxtapid)
	Ceritinib (Zykadia)	**Mifepristone** (Korlym)
	Cobicistat (Stribild)	**Nelfinavir** (Viracept)
	Conivaptan (Vaprisol)	**Ritonavir** (Norvir)
	Cyclosporine (Neoral)	**Saquinavir** (Invirase)
	Darunavir (Prezista)	**Telaprevir** (Incivek)
	Delavirdine (Rescriptor)	**Verapamil** (Isoptin)

COMMENTS: Ranolazine is metabolized primarily by CYP3A4, and inhibitors of this isozyme increase the serum concentrations of ranolazine. The product information states that ranolazine is contraindicated with potent or moderately potent CYP3A4 inhibitors. Theoretically, such drugs could increase the risk of ranolazine-induced QTc prolongation and ventricular arrhythmias. Because **amiodarone** inhibits CYP3A4 and also intrinsically prolongs the QTc interval, it would be wise to avoid combining it with ranolazine (**Class 1**).

CLASS 2: USE ONLY IF BENEFIT FELT TO OUTWEIGH RISK
- *Use Alternative*: Use an alternative to the enzyme inhibitor if possible.
  Calcium channel blockers: Calcium channel blockers other than diltiazem and verapamil are unlikely to inhibit CYP3A4.
  Grapefruit: Orange juice does not appear to inhibit CYP3A4.
- *Circumvent/Minimize*: Consider reducing the dose of the ranolazine if enzyme inhibitors are coadministered.
- *Monitor:* If the combination is used, the primary concern is QTc prolongation. Monitor the ECG and advise the patient to report any episodes of dizziness or syncope.

OBJECT DRUGS	PRECIPITANT DRUGS
Rifabutin (Mycobutin)	**Antidepressants:**
	Fluvoxamine (Luvox)
	Nefazodone

COMMENTS: Rifabutin serum concentrations can be markedly increased by CYP3A4 inhibitors; toxicity is often manifested by uveitis but rash, bone marrow suppression, and increased hepatic enzymes can also occur.

CLASS 2: USE ONLY IF BENEFIT FELT TO OUTWEIGH RISK
- *Use Alternative*: **Sertraline** (Zoloft), **citalopram** (Celexa), **escitalopram** (Lexapro), **venlafaxine** (Effexor), and **paroxetine** (Paxil) appear less likely to inhibit CYP3A4. **Fluoxetine** (Prozac) appears to be a weak inhibitor of CYP3A4.
- *Circumvent/Minimize*: Rifabutin dose may require reduction if used with CYP3A4 inhibitors.
- *Monitor*: If CYP3A4 inhibitors are used with rifabutin, monitor for rifabutin toxicity.

OBJECT DRUGS	PRECIPITANT DRUGS	
Rifabutin (Mycobutin)	**Antimicrobials:**	
	Ciprofloxacin (Cipro)	**Posaconazole** (Noxafil)
	Clarithromycin (Biaxin)	**Quinupristin** (Synercid)
	Erythromycin (E-Mycin)	**Telithromycin** (Ketek)
	Fluconazole (Diflucan)	**Troleandomycin** (TAO)
	Itraconazole (Sporanox)	**Voriconazole** (Vfend)
	Ketoconazole (Nizoral)	

COMMENTS: Rifabutin serum concentrations can be markedly increased by CYP3A4 inhibitors; toxicity is often manifested by uveitis but rash, bone marrow suppression, and increased hepatic enzymes can also occur. Also, rifabutin may substantially reduce plasma concentrations of clarithromycin, and probably also most of the other antimicrobials listed.

CLASS 2: USE ONLY IF BENEFIT FELT TO OUTWEIGH RISK
- *Use Alternative*:
  Azole Antifungals: Itraconazole and ketoconazole are potent inhibitors of CYP3A4; fluconazole appears weaker, but in larger doses it also inhibits CYP3A4. **Terbinafine** (Lamisil) does not appear to affect CYP3A4, and would not be expected to interact with rifabutin.

Macrolide Antibiotics: Unlike erythromycin, clarithromycin and troleandomycin, **azithromycin** (Zithromax) and **dirithromycin*** do not appear to inhibit CYP3A4. (*not available in US)
Telithromycin: The use of **azithromycin** (Zithromax) or a quinolone antibiotic other than ciprofloxacin could be considered.
- *Circumvent/Minimize:* Rifabutin dose may require reduction if used with CYP3A4 inhibitors.
- *Monitor:* If CYP3A4 inhibitors are used with rifabutin, monitor for rifabutin toxicity, especially uveitis.

OBJECT DRUGS	PRECIPITANT DRUGS	
Rifabutin (Mycobutin)	**Enzyme Inhibitors:**	
	Amiodarone (Cordarone)	**Diltiazem** (Cardizem)
	Amprenavir (Agenerase)	**Dronedarone** (Multaq)
	Aprepitant (Emend)	**Grapefruit**
	Atazanavir (Reyataz)	**Indinavir** (Crixivan)
	Boceprevir (Victrelis)	**Lomitapide** (Juxtapid)
	Ceritinib (Zykadia)	**Mifepristone** (Korlym)
	Cobicistat (Stribild)	**Nelfinavir** (Viracept)
	Conivaptan (Vaprisol)	**Ritonavir** (Norvir)
	Cyclosporine (Neoral)	**Saquinavir** (Invirase)
	Darunavir (Prezista)	**Telaprevir** (Incivek)
	Delavirdine (Rescriptor)	**Verapamil** (Isoptin)

COMMENTS: Rifabutin serum concentrations can be markedly increased by CYP3A4 inhibitors; toxicity is often manifested by uveitis but rash, bone marrow suppression, and increased hepatic enzymes can also occur. Also, the plasma concentrations of some of the enzyme inhibitors listed above (e.g., cyclosporine, diltiazem, verapamil) are likely to be substantially reduced due to the ability of rifabutin to act as an enzyme inducer.

CLASS 2: USE ONLY IF BENEFIT FELT TO OUTWEIGH RISK
- *Use Alternative:*
  Enzyme Inhibitor: Use an alternative to the enzyme inhibitor if possible.
  Calcium Channel Blockers: Calcium channel blockers other than diltiazem and verapamil are unlikely to inhibit the metabolism of rifabutin. But most calcium channel blockers are highly susceptible to enzyme induction, so rifabutin is likely to substantially reduce their plasma concentrations.
  Grapefruit: Orange juice does not appear to inhibit CYP3A4.
- *Circumvent/Minimize:* Rifabutin dose may require reduction if used with CYP3A4 inhibitors. In patients on ritonavir, the use of rifabutin once or twice weekly has been successful in some patients.
- *Monitor:* If CYP3A4 inhibitors are used with rifabutin, monitor for rifabutin toxicity.

OBJECT DRUGS	PRECIPITANT DRUGS
Tamoxifen (Nolvadex)	**Antidepressants:**
	Bupropion (Wellbutrin)
	Duloxetine (Cymbalta)
	Fluoxetine (Prozac)
	Paroxetine (Paxil)

COMMENTS: Tamoxifen is a prodrug that is converted to active metabolites by CYP2D6. Evidence from studies in patients with breast cancer have suggested that patients on potent CYP2D6 inhibitors have reduced concentrations of active tamoxifen metabolites, and reduced survival. People with "normal" CYP2D6 activity ("Rapid Metabolizers") would be at the greatest risk of these interactions. There is recent evidence suggesting that CYP2D6 activity may not be as important as earlier thought, but given the potential severity of the interaction it would be prudent to avoid CYP2D6 inhibitors in patients on tamoxifen until conclusive evidence is available. Many antidepressants have little effect on CYP2D6 (see below).

CLASS 2: USE ONLY IF BENEFIT FELT TO OUTWEIGH RISK
- *Use Alternative:*
  Antidepressant: Given the severity of the potential interaction, every effort should be made to avoid the above antidepressants in patients receiving tamoxifen. Alternative antidepressants have less effect on CYP2D6: **citalopram** (Celexa), **desvenlafaxine** (Pristiq), **escitalopram** (Lexapro), and **sertraline** (Zoloft), are weak inhibitors of CYP2D6, and **fluvoxamine** and **venlafaxine** (Effexor) have little or no effect on CYP2D6.
- *Monitor:* If CYP2D6 inhibitors are used with tamoxifen, be alert for evidence of reduced tamoxifen effect.

OBJECT DRUGS	PRECIPITANT DRUGS
Tamoxifen (Nolvadex)	**Enzyme Inhibitors (CYP2D6):**

Abiraterone (Zytiga)	**Mirabegron** (Myrbetriq)
Amiodarone (Cordarone)	**Propafenone** (Rythmol)
Cimetidine (Tagamet)	**Propoxyphene***
Cinacalcet (Sensipar)	**Quinidine** (Quinidex)
Clobazam (Onfi)	**Ritonavir** (Norvir)
Diphenhydramine (Benadryl)	**Terbinafine** (Lamisil)
Haloperidol (Haldol)	**Thioridazine** (Mellaril)

* Propoxyphene (Darvon) was withdrawn from the US market.

COMMENTS: Tamoxifen is a prodrug that is converted to active metabolites by CYP2D6. Evidence from studies in patients with breast cancer have suggested that patients on potent CYP2D6 inhibitors have reduced concentrations of active tamoxifen metabolites, and reduced survival. People with "normal" CYP2D6 activity ("Rapid Metabolizers") would be at the greatest risk of these interactions. There is recent evidence suggesting that CYP2D6 activity may not be as important as earlier thought, but given the potential severity of the interaction it would be prudent to avoid CYP2D6 inhibitors in patients on tamoxifen until conclusive evidence is available. Note that because terbinafine has an extraordinarily long terminal half-life, the inhibitory effect of terbinafine on CYP2D6 may last for many weeks after terbinafine is discontinued.

CLASS 2: USE ONLY IF BENEFIT FELT TO OUTWEIGH RISK
- *Use Alternative*:
  Cimetidine: **Famotidine** (Pepcid), **nizatidine** (Axid), and **ranitidine** (Zantac) have minimal effects on drug metabolism.
  Diphenhydramine: Other antihistamines such as **desloratadine** (Clarinex), **fexofenadine** (Allegra), **loratadine** Claritin), and **cetirizine** (Zyrtec) are not known to inhibit CYP2D6.
- *Monitor*: If CYP2D6 inhibitors are used with tamoxifen, be alert for evidence of reduced tamoxifen effect.

OBJECT DRUGS	PRECIPITANT DRUGS
Tamoxifen (Nolvadex)	**Enzyme Inducers:**

Barbiturates	**Phenytoin** (Dilantin)
Carbamazepine (Tegretol)	**Primidone** (Mysoline)
Dabrafenib (Tafinlar)	**Rifabutin** (Mycobutin)
Efavirenz (Sustiva)	**Rifampin** (Rifadin)
Lumacaftor (Orkambi)	**Rifapentine** (Priftin)
Nevirapine (Viramune)	**St. John's wort**
Oxcarbazepine (Trileptal)	

COMMENTS: In patients receiving tamoxifen a trial of rifampin substantially reduced plasma concentrations of tamoxifen and several of its metabolites, including the putative active metabolite, endoxifen. The study was stopped early due concerns that tamoxifen would be rendered ineffective by rifampin. Little is known regarding the effect of other enzyme inducers on tamoxifen, but consider the possibility of a similar interaction. Theoretically, enzyme inducers other than rifampin may have somewhat less effect on tamoxifen.

CLASS 2: USE ONLY IF BENEFIT FELT TO OUTWEIGH RISK
- *Use Alternative:* If available, use a drug that is not an enzyme inducer.
  St. John's wort: Given the limited evidence of efficacy, St. John's wort should generally be avoided in patients taking tamoxifen.
- *Monitor*: If the enzyme inducer must be given with tamoxifen, it would be prudent to monitor tamoxifen and metabolite concentrations (if available). Keep in mind that enzyme induction is usually gradual and may take days to weeks for onset and offset, depending on the specific inducer.

OBJECT DRUGS	PRECIPITANT DRUGS
Tetracyclines:	**Absorption Inhibitors:**
Demeclocycline (Declomycin)	**Antacids**
Doxycycline (Vibramycin)	**Bismuth** (Pepto Bismol)
Minocycline (Minocin)	**Didanosine** (Videx)
Oxytetracycline	**Iron Products**
Tetracycline	**Sucralfate** (Carafate)
	Zinc

COMMENTS: The absorption of tetracyclines may be reduced by agents containing cations such as aluminum, magnesium, and to a lesser extent, iron. Doxycycline may be less susceptible to these interactions than other tetracyclines, and does not appear to be affected significantly by iron.

CLASS 3: ASSESS RISK & TAKE ACTION IF NECESSARY
- *Circumvent/Minimize*: Give the tetracycline 2 hours before or 6 hours after the absorption inhibitor to minimize the interaction. Enteric coated didanosine (Videx EC) does not appear to interact.
- *Monitor*: Watch for reduced tetracycline efficacy in patients taking absorption inhibitors.

OBJECT DRUGS	PRECIPITANT DRUGS	
Theophylline	**Enzyme Inducers:**	
	Barbiturates	**Nevirapine** (Viramune)
	Bosentan (Tracleer)	**Oxcarbazepine** (Trileptal)
	Carbamazepine (Tegretol)	**Phenytoin** (Dilantin)
	Dabrafenib (Tafinlar)	**Primidone** (Mysoline)
	Dexamethasone (Decadron)	**Rifabutin** (Mycobutin)
	Efavirenz (Sustiva)	**Rifampin** (Rifadin)
	Griseofulvin	**Rifapentine** (Priftin)
	Lumacaftor (Orkambi)	**St. John's wort**

COMMENTS: Enzyme inducers enhance the metabolism of theophylline by CYP3A4 and probably also CYP1A2, thus reducing theophylline serum concentrations. Higher than usual theophylline doses may be needed in the presence of an enzyme inducer. Accordingly, serious theophylline toxicity has been reported following discontinuation of an enzyme inducer in patients stabilized on theophylline.

CLASS 3: ASSESS RISK & TAKE ACTION IF NECESSARY
- *Monitor*: Monitor for altered theophylline serum concentrations if an enzyme inducer is initiated, discontinued, or changed in dosage.

OBJECT DRUGS	PRECIPITANT DRUGS
Theophylline	Fluvoxamine (Luvox)

COMMENTS: Theophylline is metabolized by CYP1A2 and to a lesser extent CYP3A4. Fluvoxamine is a potent inhibitor of CYP1A2, and may produce dramatic increases in theophylline plasma concentrations; theophylline toxicity is likely to occur.

CLASS 2: USE ONLY IF BENEFIT FELT TO OUTWEIGH RISK
- *Use Alternative*: Sertraline (Zoloft), **fluoxetine** (Prozac), **venlafaxine** (Effexor), **paroxetine** (Paxil), **citalopram** (Celexa), and **escitalopram** (Lexapro) are not known to inhibit CYP1A2. **Nefazodone** is a potent inhibitor of CYP3A4, and may increase theophylline concentrations, but probably to a lesser extent than fluvoxamine.
- *Monitor*: Monitor for altered theophylline response if a CYP1A2 inhibitor is initiated, discontinued, or the dose is changed. Evidence of theophylline toxicity includes nausea, vomiting, diarrhea, restlessness, irritability, and insomnia. Higher serum levels can result in cardiac arrhythmias or seizures.

OBJECT DRUGS	PRECIPITANT DRUGS	
Theophylline	**Antimicrobials:**	
	Ciprofloxacin (Cipro)	**Erythromycin** (E-Mycin)
	Clarithromycin (Biaxin)	**Troleandomycin** (TAO)
	Enoxacin (Penetrex)	

COMMENTS: Theophylline is metabolized by CYP1A2 and to a lesser extent CYP3A4. Inhibitors of these isozymes can increase theophylline serum concentrations; some patients may develop theophylline toxicity. Ciprofloxacin and especially enoxacin are strong inhibitors of CYP1A2, and can produce serious theophylline toxicity. Clarithromycin, erythromycin, and troleandomycin usually do not increase theophylline concentrations as much, but toxicity can still occur.

CLASS 2: USE ONLY IF BENEFIT FELT TO OUTWEIGH RISK
- *Use Alternative*:
  Macrolides: Unlike erythromycin, clarithromycin and troleandomycin, **azithromycin** (Zithromax) and **dirithromycin*** do not inhibit CYP450 isozymes. (*not available in US)
  Quinolones: **Levofloxacin** (Levaquin), **lomefloxacin** (Maxaquin), **ofloxacin** (Floxin), and **moxifloxacin** (Avelox) appear to have little effect on CYP1A2 or CYP3A4.
- *Monitor*: Monitor for altered theophylline response if a CYP1A2 inhibitor is initiated, discontinue, or the dose is changed. Evidence of theophylline toxicity includes nausea, vomiting, diarrhea, restlessness, irritability, and insomnia. Higher serum concentrations can result in cardiac arrhythmias or seizures.

OBJECT DRUGS	PRECIPITANT DRUGS	
Theophylline	**Enzyme Inhibitors:**	
	Atazanavir (Reyataz)	**Deferasirox** (Exjade)
	Cimetidine (Tagamet)	**Tacrine** (Cognex)
	Disulfiram (Antabuse)	**Thiabendazole** (Mintezol)
	Mexiletine (Mexitil)	**Ticlopidine** (Ticlid)
	Pentoxifylline (Trental)	**Zileuton** (Zyflo)

COMMENTS: Inhibitors of CYP1A2 (and to a lesser extent CYP3A4) may increase serum theophylline concentrations; some patients may develop theophylline toxicity. These inhibitors appear to have less risk of serious theophylline toxicity than the Class 2 theophylline drug interactions above.

CLASS 3: ASSESS RISK & TAKE ACTION IF NECESSARY
- *Consider Alternative*: Use an alternative to the enzyme inhibitor if possible.
  Cimetidine: Although the cimetidine-theophylline interaction is usually modest, an alternative is preferable. **Famotidine** (Pepcid), **nizatidine** (Axid), and **ranitidine** (Zantac) have minimal effects on drug metabolism.
- *Monitor*: Monitor for altered theophylline response if a CYP1A2 inhibitor is initiated, discontinued, or the dose is changed. Evidence of theophylline toxicity includes nausea, vomiting, diarrhea, restlessness, irritability, and insomnia. Higher serum concentrations can result in cardiac arrhythmias or seizures.

OBJECT DRUGS	PRECIPITANT DRUGS	
Thiazide Diuretics	**SSRI and SNRI:**	
	Citalopram (Celexa)	Levomilnacipran (Fetzima)
	Clomipramine (Anafranil)	Milnacipran (Savella)
	Desvenlafaxine (Pristiq)	Paroxetine (Paxil)
	Duloxetine (Cymbalta)	Sertraline (Zoloft)
	Escitalopram (Lexapro)	Venlafaxine (Effexor)
	Fluoxetine (Prozac)	Vilazodone (Viibryd)
	Fluvoxamine (Luvox)	Vortioxetine (Brintellix)
	Imipramine (Tofranil)	

COMMENTS: Selective serotonin reuptake inhibitors (SSRI) and selective serotonin/norepinephrine reuptake inhibitors (SNRI) have been reported to cause syndrome of inappropriate antidiuretic hormone (SIADH) with hyponatremia. Thiazide diuretics increase sodium excretion, and can have additive hyponatremic effects.

CLASS 3: ASSESS RISK & TAKE ACTION IF NECESSARY
- *Consider Alternative*:
  Antidepressants: Some evidence suggests that **mirtazapine** (Remeron) is less likely to cause hyponatremia, but more evidence is needed.
- *Monitor*: Monitor for symptoms of hyponatremia: confusion, disorientation, nausea, headache, weakness, fatigue, muscle cramps. If the hyponatremia is severe, it can lead to seizures, coma and death. In predisposed patients such as elderly women it may be prudent to measure baseline serum sodium and again a week or so after the second drug was started. Hyponatremia usually occurs within 2 to 3 weeks of starting therapy of adding the second drug.

OBJECT DRUGS	PRECIPITANT DRUGS
Thioridazine (Mellaril)	**Drugs That Inhibit CYP2D6 and Prolong the QT Interval:**
	Amiodarone (Cordarone)
	Dronedarone (Multaq)
	Haloperidol (Haldol)
	Lumefantrine (Coartem)
	Quinidine (Quinidex)
	Ranolazine (Ranexa)

COMMENTS: Thioridazine can prolong the QT interval in a dose-dependent manner. Drugs that inhibit the cytochrome P450 isozymes involved in thioridazine metabolism (primarily CYP2D6) may increase the risk of ventricular arrhythmias such as torsades de pointes. Amiodarone and quinidine are strong inhibitors of CYP2D6, and also individually prolong the QT interval. Hence, the risk of serious arrhythmias is likely to be substantially increased. The product information for thioridazine states that it is contraindicated with known CYP2D6 inhibitors or drugs that increase the QT interval.

CLASS 1: AVOID COMBINATION
- *Avoid*: Avoid the use of these drugs in patients receiving thioridazine.
- *Use Alternative:*
  Thioridazine: Most other phenothiazines produce less QT prolongation than thioridazine. **Pimozide** (Orap) can substantially prolong the QT interval and would not be a suitable substitute for thioridazine.
  Antiarrhythmics: It may be difficult to find an alternative antiarrhythmic that can be used safely with thioridazine. Several other antiarrhythmics such as **disopyramide** (Norpace), **procainamide** (Pronestyl), and **sotalol** (Betapace) can prolong the QT interval, and should be used only with extreme caution with thioridazine.
- *Monitor*: If combined therapy is necessary, monitor carefully for signs of delayed ventricular repolarization (prolonged QT interval) and symptoms of torsades de pointes including palpitations and syncope.

OBJECT DRUGS	PRECIPITANT DRUGS	
Thioridazine (Mellaril)	**Enzyme Inhibitors (CYP2D6):**	
	Abiraterone (Zytiga)	Fluoxetine (Prozac)
	Bupropion (Wellbutrin)	Fluvoxamine (Luvox)
	Chloroquine	Mirabegron (Myrbetriq)
	Cimetidine (Tagamet)	Paroxetine (Paxil)
	Cinacalcet (Sensipar)	Propoxyphene*
	Clobazam (Onfi)	Ritonavir (Norvir)
	Diphenhydramine (Benadryl)	Terbinafine (Lamisil)
	Duloxetine (Cymbalta)	

* Propoxyphene (Darvon) was withdrawn from the US market.

COMMENTS: Thioridazine can prolong the QT interval. Inhibitors of CYP2D6 may increase the risk of ventricular arrhythmias such as torsades de pointes. The product information for thioridazine states that concurrent use with known CYP2D6 inhibitors (or fluvoxamine) is contraindicated. Note that because terbinafine has an extraordinarily long terminal half-life, the inhibitory effect of terbinafine on CYP2D6 may last for many weeks after terbinafine is discontinued.

CLASS 2: USE ONLY IF BENEFIT FELT TO OUTWEIGH RISK
- *Use Alternative:* Use an alternative to the enzyme inhibitor if possible.
  Antidepressants: Citalopram (Celexa), **escitalopram** (Lexapro), **sertraline** (Zoloft), and **desvenlafaxine** (Pristiq), **venlafaxine** (Effexor) have less effect on CYP2D6 than fluoxetine and paroxetine, and would not be expected to have a large effect on thioridazine metabolism.
  Cimetidine: **Famotidine** (Pepcid), **nizatidine** (Axid), and **ranitidine** (Zantac) have no known effects on CYP2D6 activity.
  Thioridazine: Most other phenothiazines produce less QT prolongation than thioridazine. **Pimozide** (Orap) can substantially prolong the QT interval and would not be a suitable substitute for thioridazine.
- *Monitor:* If combined therapy is necessary, monitor carefully for signs of delayed ventricular repolarization (prolonged QT interval) and symptoms of torsades de pointes including palpitations and syncope.

OBJECT DRUGS	PRECIPITANT DRUGS	
Thyroid:	**Binding Agents:**	
Levothyroxine (Synthroid)	Antacids	Iron Products
Liothyronine (Cytomel)	Cholestyramine (Questran)	Lanthanum Carbonate (Fosrenol)
Liotrix (Thyrolar)	Colesevelam (WelChol)	Sevelamer (Renagel)
Thyroid USP	Colestipol (Colestid)	Sucralfate (Carafate)

COMMENTS: These binding agents may inhibit thyroid hormone absorption if given concurrently. The reduction in thyroid bioavailability can be marked; in one study colesevelam reduced thyroxine absorption by 96%. There is a large variability in the magnitude of this interaction on circulating thyroid hormones from one person to another, however, probably because some people on thyroid have some residual thyroid function. Limited evidence suggests that thyroxine absorption may also be inhibited by **ciprofloxacin** (Cipro), **caffeine**, and **sertraline** (Zoloft), but more evidence is needed to assess the clinical importance of these interactions.

CLASS 3: ASSESS RISK & TAKE ACTION IF NECESSARY
- *Circumvent/Minimize:* Minimize interactions by giving thyroid 2 hours before or 6 hours after the binding agent; keep a constant interval between doses of thyroid and binding agents. Some reduction in thyroid levels may still occur due to enterohepatic circulation of thyroxine.
- *Monitor:* Monitor If thyroid hormones are administered with binding agents, monitor for reduced thyroid effect.

OBJECT DRUGS	PRECIPITANT DRUGS	
Tizanidine (Zanaflex)	**Enzyme Inhibitors:**	
	Atazanavir (Reyataz)	**Fluvoxamine** (Luvox)
	Cimetidine (Tagamet)	**Mexiletine** (Mexitil)
	Ciprofloxacin (Cipro)	**Tacrine** (Cognex)
	Enoxacin (Penetrex)	**Zileuton** (Zyflo)
	Ethinyl Estradiol	

COMMENTS: Potent CYP1A2 inhibitors such as fluvoxamine and ciprofloxacin can produce dramatic increases in tizanidine plasma concentrations; tizanidine toxicity is likely (eg, hypotension, CHS depression). Other CYP1A2 inhibitors would generally have less effect on tizanidine, but it would be prudent to avoid the combinations when possible. For example, oral contraceptives are normally considered only moderate inhibitors of CYP1A2, but a product containing ethinyl estradiol and gestodene produced large increases in tizanidine plasma concentrations.

MANAGEMENT CLASS 2: USE ONLY IF BENEFIT FELT TO OUTWEIGH RISK
[CIPROFLOXACIN, ENOXACIN, FLUVOXAMINE]
- *Use Alternative*: Given the magnitude of the increase in tizanidine plasma concentrations, it would be prudent to avoid these combinations.
  Fluvoxamine: **Sertraline** (Zoloft), **fluoxetine** (Prozac), **venlafaxine** (Effexor), **paroxetine** (Paxil), **citalopram** (Celexa), and **escitalopram** (Lexapro) are not known to inhibit CYP1A2.
  Fluoroquinolones: **Gemifloxacin** (Factive), **levofloxacin** (Levaquin), **lomefloxacin** (Maxaquin), **moxifloxacin** (Avelox), **norfloxacin** (Noroxin), and **ofloxacin** (Floxin) appear to have little effect on CYP1A2.
- *Monitor*: If the combination is used, monitor for evidence of tizanidine toxicity such as hypotension and excessive CNS depression.

MANAGEMENT CLASS 3: ASSESS RISK AND TAKE ACTION IF NECESSARY
[ATAZANAVIR, CIMETIDINE, ETHINYL ESTRADIOL, MEXILETINE, TACRINE, ZILEUTON]
- *Consider Alternative:* If available, use a drug that is not an inhibitor of CYP1A2.
  Cimetidine: **Famotidine** (Pepcid), **nizatidine** (Axid), and **ranitidine** (Zantac) have no known effects on CYP1A2 activity.
- *Monitor:* If the combination is used, monitor for evidence of tizanidine toxicity such as hypotension and excessive CNS depression.

OBJECT DRUGS	PRECIPITANT DRUGS
Trimethoprim (Bactrim, Septra)	**Angiotensin Receptor Blockers:**
	Azilsartan (Edarbi)
	Candesartan (Atacand)
	Eprosartan (Teveten)
	Irbesartan (Avapro)
	Losartan (Cozaar)
	Olmesartan (Benicar)
	Telmisartan (Micardis)
	Valsartan (Diovan)

COMMENTS: Trimethoprim alone often produces modest increases in serum potassium, and hyperkalemia can occur when it is combined with other drugs that increase potassium such as angiotensin receptor blockers (ARBs). Hospitalizations for hyperkalemia are substantially higher in patients on ARBs who take trimethoprim versus amoxicillin, for example. The risk may be increased in the presence of one or more predisposing factors such as significant renal impairment, severe diabetes, potassium supplements, high potassium diet, advanced age or additional drugs that can increase potassium such as **ACE inhibitors, drospirenone** (Yasmin), **heparins, nonselective beta-blockers, NSAIDs, COX-2 inhibitors, cyclosporine, tacrolimus, succinylcholine, pentamidine,** and **potassium-containing salt substitutes**.

CLASS 2: USE ONLY IF BENEFIT FELT TO OUTWEIGH RISK
- *Use Alternative:* If possible use an antibiotic other than trimethoprim.
- *Monitor:* If trimethoprim is used in patients on ARBs, monitor serum potassium concentrations, especially in patients with predisposing factors such as renal disease, diabetes, and advanced age.

OBJECT DRUGS	PRECIPITANT DRUGS	
Trimethoprim (Bactrim, Septra)	**ACE inhibitors:**	
	Benazepril (Lotensin)	**Moexipril** (Univasc)
	Captopril (Capoten)	**Perindopril** (Aceon)
	Enalapril (Vasotec)	**Quinapril** (Accupril)
	Fosinopril (Monopril)	**Ramipril** (Altace)
	Lisinopril (Prinivil)	**Trandolapril** (Mavik)

COMMENTS: Trimethoprim alone often produces modest increases in serum potassium, and hyperkalemia can occur when it is combined with other drugs that increase potassium such as ACE Inhibitors (ACEI). Hospitalizations for hyperkalemia are substantially higher in patients on ACEI who take trimethoprim versus amoxicillin, for example. The risk may be increased in the presence of one or more predisposing factors such as significant renal impairment, severe diabetes, potassium supplements, high potassium diet, advanced age or additional drugs that can increase potassium such as **drospirenone** (Yasmin), **heparins, nonselective beta-blockers, NSAIDs, COX-2 inhibitors, angiotensin receptor blockers, cyclosporine, tacrolimus, succinylcholine, pentamidine,** and **potassium-containing salt substitutes.**

CLASS 2: USE ONLY IF BENEFIT FELT TO OUTWEIGH RISK
- *Use Alternative:* If possible use an antibiotic other than trimethoprim.
- *Monitor:* If trimethoprim is used in patients on ACEI, monitor serum potassium concentrations, especially in patients with predisposing factors such as renal disease, diabetes, and advanced age.

OBJECT DRUGS	PRECIPITANT DRUGS
Trimethoprim (Bactrim, Septra)	**Potassium-sparing diuretics:**
	Amiloride (Midamor)
	Eplerenone (Inspra)
	Spironolactone (Aldactone)
	Triamterene (Dyrenium)

COMMENTS: Trimethoprim alone often produces modest increases in serum potassium, and hyperkalemia can occur when it is combined with other drugs that increase potassium such as potassium-sparing diuretics. Hospitalizations for hyperkalemia are substantially higher in patients on spironolactone who take trimethoprim versus amoxicillin, for example. The risk may be increased in the presence of one or more predisposing factors such as significant renal impairment, severe diabetes, potassium supplements, high potassium diet, advanced age or additional drugs that can increase potassium such as **drospirenone** (Yasmin), **heparins, nonselective beta-blockers, NSAIDs, COX-2 inhibitors, ACE inhibitors, angiotensin receptor blockers, cyclosporine, tacrolimus, succinylcholine, pentamidine,** and **potassium-containing salt substitutes.**

CLASS 2: USE ONLY IF BENEFIT FELT TO OUTWEIGH RISK
- *Use Alternative:* If possible use an antibiotic other than trimethoprim.
- *Monitor:* If trimethoprim is used in patients on potassium-sparing diuretics, monitor serum potassium concentrations, especially in patients with predisposing factors such as renal disease, diabetes, and advanced age.

OBJECT DRUGS	PRECIPITANT DRUGS
Valproic Acid (Depakene)	**Carbapenem Antibiotics:**
	Doripenem (Doribax)
	Ertapenem (Invanz)
	Imipenem (Primaxin)
	Meropenem (Merrem)

COMMENTS: The administration of carbapenem antibiotics has been noted to markedly reduce the plasma concentrations of valproic acid. Reduction in seizure control may occur.

CLASS 3: ASSESS RISK & TAKE ACTION IF NECESSARY
- *Consider Alternative:* If possible, consider an alternative antibiotic to a carbapenem in patients taking valproic acid.
- *Monitor:* Monitor for altered valproic acid plasma concentrations and response if a carbapenem antibiotic is initiated, discontinued, or changed in dosage.

OBJECT DRUGS	PRECIPITANT DRUGS
Valproic Acid (Depakene)	Topiramate (Topamax)

COMMENTS: Valproic acid often causes an asymptomatic increase in blood ammonia, but occasionally can cause severe hyperammonemic encephalopathy. There are many case reports suggesting that concurrent administration of topiramate and valproic acid increases the risk of encephalopathy. A study also found cognitive dysfunction in some patients when topiramate was added to valproic acid therapy. Most of the symptoms are behavioral or neurologic, but severe cases can be life-threatening. The mechanism for the interaction is not clear, but may involve additive effects on blood ammonia as well as other pharmacodynamic effects. Some evidence suggests that concurrent use of phenobarbital increases the risk of encephalopathy due to valproic acid plus topiramate. Valproic acid and topiramate do not appear to have significant pharmacokinetic interactions with each other.

CLASS 3: ASSESS RISK & TAKE ACTION IF NECESSARY
- *Consider Alternative*: In patients receiving valproic acid, consider using an alternative to topiramate, especially if the patient has other factors that may predispose to encephalopathy which may include concurrent phenobarbital therapy, pre-existing chronic encephalopathy, and febrile states.
- *Monitor*: If the combination is used, it is imperative that the patient and/or caregivers are alert for evidence of encephalopathy, such as confusion, memory impairment, drowsiness, lethargy, slow speech, irritability, sleep disturbances, motor impairment, increased seizure frequency, and hypothermia. Diagnosis may be problematic if the patient displays symptoms that mimic the disorder for which he or she has received the valproate. Prompt discontinuation of the valproic acid is usually followed by resolution of the symptoms, sometimes within the first day or two.

OBJECT DRUGS	PRECIPITANT DRUGS	
Vinca Alkaloids:	**Antimicrobials:**	
Vinblastine (Velban)	**Ciprofloxacin** (Cipro)	**Posaconazole** (Noxafil)
Vincristine (Oncovin)	**Clarithromycin** (Biaxin)	**Quinupristin** (Synercid)
Vinorelbine (Navelbine)	**Erythromycin** (E-Mycin)	**Telithromycin** (Ketek)
	Fluconazole (Diflucan)	**Troleandomycin** (TAO)
	Itraconazole (Sporanox)	**Voriconazole** (Vfend)
	Ketoconazole (Nizoral)	

COMMENTS: Vinca alkaloids appear to be metabolized by CYP3A4, and reports have described severe toxicity in patients receiving concurrent therapy with CYP3A4 inhibitors. Assume that all CYP3A4 inhibitors interact until proved otherwise. P-glycoprotein inhibition may also be involved in these interactions.

CLASS 2: USE ONLY IF BENEFIT FELT TO OUTWEIGH RISK
- *Use Alternative*:
  Azole Antifungals: Itraconazole and ketoconazole are potent inhibitors of CYP3A4; fluconazole appears weaker, but in larger doses it also inhibits CYP3A4. **Terbinafine** (Lamisil) does not appear to affect CYP3A4, and would not be expected to interact with vinca alkaloids.
  Macrolide Antibiotics: Unlike erythromycin, clarithromycin and troleandomycin, **azithromycin** (Zithromax) and **dirithromycin*** do not appear to inhibit CYP3A4. (*not available in US)
  Telithromycin: The use of azithromycin (Zithromax) or a quinolone antibiotic other than ciprofloxacin could be considered.
- *Monitor*: Monitor for toxicity from vincristine (primarily peripheral neuropathy symptoms: paresthesias, neuritic pain, muscle pain, constipation sometimes progressing to paralytic ileus) or vinblastine and vinorelbine (primarily bone marrow suppression).

OBJECT DRUGS	PRECIPITANT DRUGS
Vinca Alkaloids:	**Calcium Channel Blockers:**
Vinblastine (Velban)	**Diltiazem** (Cardizem)
Vincristine (Oncovin)	**Nicardipine** (Cardene)
Vinorelbine (Navelbine)	**Nifedipine** (Procardia)
	Verapamil (Isoptin)

COMMENTS: Vinca alkaloids appear to be metabolized by CYP3A4 and reports have described severe toxicity in patients receiving CYP3A4 inhibitors such as verapamil. P-glycoprotein inhibition may also be involved in these interactions.

CLASS 2: USE ONLY IF BENEFIT FELT TO OUTWEIGH RISK
- *Use Alternative*: Use an alternative to the enzyme inhibitor if possible.
  Calcium channel blockers: Calcium channel blockers other than diltiazem, nicardipine, nifedipine, and verapamil are unlikely to inhibit the metabolism of vinca alkaloids.
- *Monitor*: Monitor for toxicity from vincristine (primarily peripheral neuropathy symptoms: paresthesias, neuritic pain, muscle pain, constipation sometimes progressing to paralytic ileus) or vinblastine and vinorelbine (primarily bone marrow suppression).

OBJECT DRUGS	PRECIPITANT DRUGS	
Vinca Alkaloids:	**Enzyme Inhibitors:**	
Vinblastine (Velban)	**Amiodarone** (Cordarone)	**Dronedarone** (Multaq)
Vincristine (Oncovin)	**Amprenavir** (Agenerase)	**Fluvoxamine** (Luvox)
Vinorelbine (Navelbine)	**Aprepitant** (Emend)	**Grapefruit**
	Atazanavir (Reyataz)	**Indinavir** (Crixivan)
	Boceprevir (Victrelis)	**Lomitapide** (Juxtapid)
	Ceritinib (Zykadia)	**Mifepristone** (Korlym)
	Cobicistat (Stribild)	**Nefazodone**
	Conivaptan (Vaprisol)	**Nelfinavir** (Viracept)
	Cyclosporine (Neoral)	**Ritonavir** (Norvir)
	Darunavir (Prezista)	**Saquinavir** (Invirase)
	Delavirdine (Rescriptor)	**Telaprevir** (Incivek)

COMMENTS: Vinca alkaloids appear to be metabolized by CYP3A4 and several reports have described severe vincristine toxicity in patients receiving CYP3A4 inhibitors. P-glycoprotein inhibition may also be involved in these interactions.

CLASS 2: USE ONLY IF BENEFIT FELT TO OUTWEIGH RISK
- *Use Alternative*: Use an alternative to the enzyme inhibitor if possible.
  Antidepressants: **Sertraline** (Zoloft), **citalopram** (Celexa), **escitalopram** (Lexapro), **venlafaxine** (Effexor), and **paroxetine** (Paxil) appear less likely to inhibit CYP3A4. **Fluoxetine** (Prozac) appears to be only a weak inhibitor of CYP3A4.
  Grapefruit: Orange juice does not appear to inhibit CYP3A4.
- *Monitor*: Monitor for toxicity from vincristine (primarily peripheral neuropathy symptoms: paresthesias, neuritic pain, muscle pain, constipation sometimes progressing to paralytic ileus) or vinblastine and vinorelbine (primarily bone marrow suppression).

OBJECT DRUGS	PRECIPITANT DRUGS	
Zidovudine (Retrovir)	**Enzyme Inducers:**	
	Barbiturates	**Phenytoin** (Dilantin)
	Carbamazepine (Tegretol)	**Primidone** (Mysoline)
	Dabrafenib (Tafinlar)	**Rifabutin** (Mycobutin)
	Efavirenz (Sustiva)	**Rifampin** (Rifadin)
	Nevirapine (Viramune)	**Rifapentine** (Priftin)
	Oxcarbazepine (Trileptal)	**St. John's wort**

COMMENTS: Enzyme inducers such as rifampin and rifabutin may enhance zidovudine metabolism, thus reducing its effect. Little is known regarding the effect of other enzyme inducers on zidovudine, but consider the possibility of a similar interaction.

CLASS 3: ASSESS RISK & TAKE ACTION IF NECESSARY
* *Consider Alternative:* If available, use a drug that is not an enzyme inducer.
  St. John's wort: Given the limited evidence of efficacy, St. John's wort should generally be avoided in patients taking zidovudine.
* *Monitor:* Zidovudine dose may need to be adjusted if enzyme inducer therapy is initiated or discontinued. Keep in mind that enzyme induction is usually gradual and may take days to weeks for onset and offset, depending on the specific inducer.

OBJECT DRUGS	PRECIPITANT DRUGS
Zidovudine (Retrovir)	**Glucuronidation Inhibitors:**
	Probenecid (Benemid)
	Trimethoprim (Bactrim)
	Valproic acid (Depakene)

COMMENTS: Drugs that can inhibit glucuronidation such as probenecid, trimethoprim, and valproic acid may increase zidovudine serum concentrations, probably by inhibition of hepatic metabolism (reduced renal excretion may also be involved). Zidovudine toxicity (e.g., anemia) has been reported.

CLASS 3: ASSESS RISK & TAKE ACTION IF NECESSARY
* *Consider Alternative:* If possible use an alternative to the glucuronidation inhibitor. Some have recommended use of an alternative to the zidovudine that is not metabolized by glucuronidation. In one case substitution of **stavudine** (Zerit) for zidovudine was successful.
* *Monitor:* Zidovudine dose may need to be adjusted if these drugs are initiated, discontinued or changed in dosage. Watch for anemia in patients receiving zidovudine and valproic acid.

OBJECT DRUGS	PRECIPITANT DRUGS
Bedaquiline (Sirturo)	**Antidepressants:**
	Fluvoxamine (Luvox)
	Nefazodone

COMMENTS: Bedaquiline is a CYP3A4 substrate, and CYP3A4, inhibitors such as fluvoxamine or nefazodone may increase the risk of bedaquiline toxicity. Bedaquiline can produce hepatotoxicity and can prolong the QTc interval, thus increasing the risk of ventricular arrhythmias.

CLASS 3: ASSESS RISK & TAKE ACTION IF NECESSARY
* *Consider Alternative:* **Sertraline** (Zoloft), **venlafaxine** (Effexor), **paroxetine** (Paxil), **citalopram** (Celexa), and **escitalopram** (Lexapro) are not known to inhibit CYP3A4. **Fluoxetine** (Prozac) appears to be a weak CYP3A4 inhibitor.
* *Monitor:* If the combination is used, monitor for evidence of hepatotoxicity and monitor the ECG for evidence of QTc prolongation.

OBJECT DRUGS	PRECIPITANT DRUGS	
Bedaquiline (Sirturo)	**Antimicrobials:**	
	Ciprofloxacin (Cipro)	**Posaconazole** (Noxafil)
	Clarithromycin (Biaxin)	**Quinupristin** (Synercid)
	Erythromycin (E-Mycin)	**Telithromycin** (Ketek)
	Fluconazole (Diflucan)	**Troleandomycin** (TAO)
	Itraconazole (Sporanox)	**Voriconazole** (Vfend)
	Ketoconazole (Nizoral)	

COMMENTS: Bedaquiline is metabolized by CYP3A4 and concurrent administration of CYP3A4 inhibiting antimicrobials may increase the risk of bedaquiline toxicity. Bedaquiline can produce hepatotoxicity and can prolong the QTc interval, thus increasing the risk of ventricular arrhythmias.

CLASS 3: ASSESS RISK & TAKE ACTION IF NECESSARY
- *Consider Alternative*:
- Azole Antifungals: Itraconazole and ketoconazole are potent inhibitors of CYP3A4; fluconazole appears weaker, but in larger doses it also inhibits CYP3A4. **Terbinafine** (Lamisil) does not appear to affect CYP3A4, and would not be expected to interact with bedaquiline.
Macrolide Antibiotics: Unlike erythromycin, clarithromycin and troleandomycin, **azithromycin** (Zithromax) and **dirithromycin*** do not appear to inhibit CYP3A4. (*not available in US)
Telithromycin: The use of **azithromycin** (Zithromax) or a quinolone antibiotic other than ciprofloxacin should be considered.
- *Monitor*: If the combination is used, monitor for evidence of hepatotoxicity and monitor the ECG for evidence of QTc prolongation.

OBJECT DRUGS	PRECIPITANT DRUGS
Bedaquiline (Sirturo)	**Calcium Channel Blockers:**
	Diltiazem (Cardizem)
	Verapamil (Isoptin)

COMMENTS: Bedaquiline is a CYP3A4 substrate, and CYP3A4, inhibitors such as diltiazem and verapamil may increase the risk of bedaquiline toxicity. Bedaquiline can produce hepatotoxicity and can prolong the QTc interval, thus increasing the risk of ventricular arrhythmias.

CLASS 3: ASSESS RISK & TAKE ACTION IF NECESSARY
- *Consider Alternative*: Calcium channel blockers other than diltiazem and verapamil are unlikely to inhibit the metabolism of bedaquiline.
- *Monitor*: If the combination is used, monitor for evidence of hepatotoxicity and monitor the ECG for evidence of QTc prolongation.

OBJECT DRUGS	PRECIPITANT DRUGS	
Bedaquiline (Sirturo)	**Enzyme Inhibitors:**	
	Amiodarone (Cordarone)	**Delavirdine** (Rescriptor)
	Amprenavir (Agenerase)	**Dronedarone** (Multaq)
	Aprepitant (Emend)	**Grapefruit**
	Atazanavir (Reyataz)	**Indinavir** (Crixivan)
	Boceprevir (Victrelis)	**Lomitapide** (Juxtapid)
	Cimetidine (Tagamet)	**Mifepristone** (Korlym)
	Cobicistat (Stribild)	**Nelfinavir** (Viracept)
	Conivaptan (Vaprisol)	**Ritonavir** (Norvir)
	Cyclosporine (Neoral)	**Saquinavir** (Invirase)
	Darunavir (Prezista)	**Telaprevir** (Incivek)

COMMENTS: Bedaquiline is metabolized by CYP3A4 and concurrent administration with CYP3A4 inhibitors may increase the risk of bedaquiline toxicity. Bedaquiline can produce hepatotoxicity and can prolong the QTc interval, thus increasing the risk of ventricular arrhythmias.

CLASS 3: ASSESS RISK & TAKE ACTION IF NECESSARY
- *Consider Alternative*:
Cimetidine: **Famotidine** (Pepcid), **nizatidine** (Axid), and **ranitidine** (Zantac) have minimal effects on drug metabolism.
Grapefruit: Orange juice does not appear to inhibit CYP3A4.
- *Monitor*: If bedaquiline is used with CYP3A4 inhibitors, monitor for evidence of hepatotoxicity and monitor the ECG for evidence of QTc prolongation.

OBJECT DRUGS	PRECIPITANT DRUGS	
Bedaquiline (Sirturo)	**Enzyme Inducers:**	
	Barbiturates	**Phenytoin** (Dilantin)
	Bosentan (Tracleer)	**Primidone** (Mysoline)
	Carbamazepine (Tegretol)	**Rifabutin** (Mycobutin)
	Dabrafenib (Tafinlar)	**Rifampin** (Rifadin)
	Dexamethasone (Decadron)	**Rifapentine** (Priftin)
	Efavirenz (Sustiva)	**St. John's wort**
	Lumacaftor (Orkambi)	
	Oxcarbazepine (Trileptal)	

COMMENTS: Bedaquiline is metabolized by CYP3A4, and enzyme inducers may substantially reduce serum bedaquiline concentrations. In one study, 3 weeks of rifampin therapy reduced bedaquiline AUC by about 50%. The product information for bedaquiline states that enzyme inducers should not be administered with bedaquiline. Although **nevirapine** (Viramune) is a CYP3A4 inducer, the manufacturer reports that 4 weeks of nevirapine 400 mg daily did not have a clinically relevant effect on bedaquiline exposure.

CLASS 2: USE ONLY IF BENEFIT FELT TO OUTWEIGH RISK
- *Use Alternative*:
  Anticonvulsants: In patients on bedaquiline it would be desirable to use anticonvulsants that are not enzyme inducers, but in many cases it may not be reasonable to change the patient's anticonvulsant regimen.
  HIV Medications. Since most antiviral medications are either inducers or inhibitors of CYP3A4, it may not be possible to avoid these interactions in most cases.
  St. John's wort: Given the questionable benefit of St. John's wort, it would be prudent to avoid giving it with bedaquiline.
- *Monitor*: Monitor for altered bedaquiline effect if enzyme inducers are initiated, discontinued, or changed in dosage. Adjustments in bedaquiline dosage may be necessary. Keep in mind that enzyme induction is usually gradual and may take days to weeks for onset and offset, depending on the specific inducer.

OBJECT DRUGS	PRECIPITANT DRUGS
Dolutegravir (Tivicay)	**Binding Agents:**
	Antacids
	Calcium supplements
	Iron
	Magnesium supplements
	Sucralfate (Carafate)

COMMENTS: Polyvalent cations may inhibit dolutegravir absorption. The reduction in dolutegravir bioavailability can be substantial; in one study magnesium-aluminum hydroxide antacid reduced dolutegravir absorption by 74%.

CLASS 3: ASSESS RISK & TAKE ACTION IF NECESSARY
- *Circumvent/Minimize*: Minimize the interaction by giving dolutegravir 2 hours before or 6 hours after the binding agent.`
- *Monitor*: If dolutegravir is administered with binding agents, monitor for reduced dolutegravir effect.

OBJECT DRUGS	PRECIPITANT DRUGS
Almotriptan (Axert)	**Antidepressants:**
Eletriptan (Relpax)	**Fluvoxamine** (Luvox)
	Nefazodone

COMMENTS: Almotriptan and eletriptan are CYP3A4 substrates, and CYP3A4 inhibitors such as fluvoxamine or nefazodone may increase the risk of toxicity. Hypertension, tachycardia or coronary vasospasm may occur if administered with CYP3A4 inhibitors.

CLASS 2: USE ONLY IF BENEFIT FELT TO OUTWEIGH RISK
- *Use Alternative*:
  Triptans: **Naratriptan** (Amerge), **Zolmitriptan** (Zomig), and **Sumatriptan** (Imitrex), are not CYP3A4 substrates.
  Antidepressants: **Sertraline** (Zoloft), **venlafaxine** (Effexor), **paroxetine** (Paxil), **citalopram** (Celexa), and **escitalopram** (Lexapro) are not known to inhibit CYP3A4. **Fluoxetine** (Prozac) appears to be a weak CYP3A4 inhibitor.
- *Monitor*: If the combination is used, monitor for evidence of vasoconstriction such as hypertension.

OBJECT DRUGS	PRECIPITANT DRUGS	
Almotriptan (Axert)	**Antimicrobials:**	
Eletriptan (Relpax)	**Ciprofloxacin** (Cipro)	**Posaconazole** (Noxafil)
	Clarithromycin (Biaxin)	**Quinupristin** (Synercid)
	Erythromycin (E-Mycin)	**Telithromycin** (Ketek)
	Fluconazole (Diflucan)	**Troleandomycin** (TAO)
	Itraconazole (Sporanox)	**Voriconazole** (Vfend)
	Ketoconazole (Nizoral)	

COMMENTS: Almotriptan and eletriptan are CYP3A4 substrates, and antimicrobials that are CYP3A4 inhibitors may increase the risk of toxicity. Hypertension, tachycardia or coronary vasospasm may occur if administered with CYP3A4 inhibitors.

CLASS 2: USE ONLY IF BENEFIT FELT TO OUTWEIGH RISK
- *Use Alternative*:
  Triptans: **Naratriptan** (Amerge), **Zolmitriptan** (Zomig), and **Sumatriptan** (Imitrex), are not CYP3A4 substrates.
  Azole Antifungals: Itraconazole and ketoconazole are potent inhibitors of CYP3A4; fluconazole appears weaker, but in larger doses it also inhibits CYP3A4. **Terbinafine** (Lamisil) does not appear to affect CYP3A4, and would not be expected to interact with the triptans.
  Macrolide Antibiotics: Unlike erythromycin, clarithromycin and troleandomycin, **azithromycin** (Zithromax) and **dirithromycin*** do not appear to inhibit CYP3A4. (*not available in US)
  Telithromycin: The use of **azithromycin** (Zithromax) or a quinolone antibiotic other than ciprofloxacin should be considered.
- *Monitor*: If the combination is used, monitor for evidence of vasoconstriction such as hypertension.

OBJECT DRUGS	PRECIPITANT DRUGS
Almotriptan (Axert)	**Calcium Channel Blockers:**
Eletriptan (Relpax)	**Diltiazem** (Cardizem)
	Verapamil (Isoptin)

COMMENTS: Almotriptan and eletriptan are CYP3A4 substrates, and CYP3A4 inhibitors such as diltiazem or verapamil may increase the risk of toxicity. Hypertension, tachycardia or coronary vasospasm may occur if administered with CYP3A4 inhibitors.

CLASS 2: USE ONLY IF BENEFIT FELT TO OUTWEIGH RISK
- *Use Alternative*:
  Triptans: **Naratriptan** (Amerge), **Zolmitriptan** (Zomig), and **Sumatriptan** (Imitrex), are not CYP3A4 substrates.
  Calcium channel blockers other than diltiazem and verapamil are unlikely to inhibit the metabolism of almotriptan and eletriptan.
- *Monitor*: If the combination is used, monitor for evidence of vasoconstriction such as hypertension.

OBJECT DRUGS	PRECIPITANT DRUGS	
Almotriptan (Axert)	**Enzyme Inhibitors:**	
Eletriptan (Relpax)	Amiodarone (Cordarone)	Delavirdine (Rescriptor)
	Amprenavir (Agenerase)	Dronedarone (Multaq)
	Aprepitant (Emend)	Grapefruit
	Atazanavir (Reyataz)	Indinavir (Crixivan)
	Boceprevir (Victrelis)	Lomitapide (Juxtapid)
	Ceritinib (Zykadia)	Mifepristone (Korlym)
	Cimetidine (Tagamet)	Nelfinavir (Viracept)
	Cobicistat (Stribild)	Ritonavir (Norvir)
	Conivaptan (Vaprisol)	Saquinavir (Invirase)
	Cyclosporine (Neoral)	Telaprevir (Incivek)
	Darunavir (Prezista)	

COMMENTS: Almotriptan and eletriptan are CYP3A4 substrates, and CYP3A4 inhibitors may increase the risk of toxicity. Hypertension, tachycardia or coronary vasospasm may occur if administered with CYP3A4 inhibitors.

CLASS 2: USE ONLY IF BENEFIT FELT TO OUTWEIGH RISK
- *Use Alternative*:
  Cimetidine: **Famotidine** (Pepcid), **nizatidine** (Axid), and **ranitidine** (Zantac) have minimal effects on drug metabolism.
  Grapefruit: Orange juice does not appear to inhibit CYP3A4.
- *Monitor:* If the combination is used, monitor for evidence of vasoconstriction such as hypertension.

OBJECT DRUGS		PRECIPITANT DRUGS
NSAIDs:		**Aldosterone Antagonists:**
Diclofenac (Voltaren)	Meclofenamate	Eplerenone (Inspra)
Diflunisal (Dolobid)	Mefenamic acid	Spironolactone (Aldactone)
Etodolac (Lodine)	Meloxicam (Mobic)	
Fenoprofen (Nalfon)	Nabumetone (Relafen)	
Flurbiprofen (Ansaid)	Naproxen (Aleve)	
Ibuprofen (Motrin)	Oxaprozin (Daypro)	
Indomethacin (Indocin)	Piroxicam (Feldene)	
Ketoprofen (Orudis)	Sulindac (Clinoril)	
Ketorolac (Toradol)	Tolmetin (Tolectin)	

COMMENTS: The concurrent use of NSAIDs with aldosterone antagonists appears to increase the risk of gastrointestinal (GI) bleeding compared to either drug used alone. Although the vast majority of patients on concurrent therapy with an NSAID and an aldosterone antagonist will not develop GI bleeding, the potential severity of the outcome (including death) suggests that the risk should be avoided if possible.

CLASS 3: ASSESS RISK & TAKE ACTION IF NECESSARY
- *Consider Alternative*:
  NSAIDs: If the NSAID is being used as an analgesic, consider using acetaminophen instead.
  Combining COX-2 inhibitors with aldosterone antagonists may increase the risk of GI bleeding over either drug alone, but the risk is probably less with COX-2 inhibitors + aldosterone antagonists than with NSAIDs + aldosterone antagonists.
- *Monitor:* Patients and health professionals should be alert for evidence of gastrointestinal bleeding if these combinations are used.

OBJECT DRUGS		PRECIPITANT DRUGS
NSAIDs or Aspirin:		**Corticosteroids:**
Diclofenac (Voltaren)	**Meclofenamate**	Cortisone (Cortone)
Diflunisal (Dolobid)	**Mefenamic acid**	Dexamethasone (Decadron)
Etodolac (Lodine)	**Meloxicam** (Mobic)	Hydrocortisone (Cortef)
Fenoprofen (Nalfon)	**Nabumetone** (Relafen)	Methylprednisolone (Medrol)
Flurbiprofen (Ansaid)	**Naproxen** (Aleve)	Prednisolone (Orapred)
Ibuprofen (Motrin)	**Oxaprozin** (Daypro)	Prednisone
Indomethacin (Indocin)	**Piroxicam** (Feldene)	Triamcinolone (Aristocort)
Ketoprofen (Orudis)	**Sulindac** (Clinoril)	
Ketorolac (Toradol)	**Tolmetin** (Tolectin)	

COMMENTS: The concurrent use of NSAIDs or aspirin (even low dose aspirin) with systemic corticosteroids appears to increase the risk of gastrointestinal (GI) bleeding compared to either drug used alone. In one study the risk appeared to be synergistic rather than additive. Although the vast majority of patients on concurrent therapy with an NSAID or aspirin with corticosteroids will not develop GI bleeding, the potential severity of the outcome (including death) suggests that the risk should be avoided if possible.

CLASS 3: ASSESS RISK & TAKE ACTION IF NECESSARY
- *Consider Alternative*:
  NSAIDs: If the NSAID is being used as an analgesic, consider using acetaminophen instead. Combining COX-2 inhibitors with corticosteroids may increase the risk of GI bleeding over either drug alone, but the risk is probably less with COX-2 inhibitors + corticosteroids than with NSAIDs + corticosteroids.
- *Monitor*: Patients and health professionals should be alert for evidence of gastrointestinal bleeding if these combinations are used.
-

OBJECT DRUGS	PRECIPITANT DRUGS
Flibanserin (Addyi)	**Antidepressants:**
	Fluvoxamine (Luvox)
	Nefazodone

COMMENTS: Flibanserin is a CYP3A4 substrate, and CYP3A4 inhibitors such as fluvoxamine or nefazodone may increase the risk of flibanserin toxicity.

CLASS 3: ASSESS RISK & TAKE ACTION IF NECESSARY
- *Consider Alternative*: **Sertraline** (Zoloft), **venlafaxine** (Effexor), **paroxetine** (Paxil), **citalopram** (Celexa), and **escitalopram** (Lexapro) are not known to inhibit CYP3A4. **Fluoxetine** (Prozac) appears to be a weak CYP3A4 inhibitor.
- *Monitor*: If flibanserin is used with CYP3A4 inhibitors, monitor for evidence of flibanserin toxicity such as hypotension, fainting, and CNS depression. Reduce flibanserin dose as needed.

OBJECT DRUGS	PRECIPITANT DRUGS	
Flibanserin (Addyi)	**Antimicrobials:**	
	Ciprofloxacin (Cipro)	**Posaconazole** (Noxafil)
	Clarithromycin (Biaxin)	**Quinupristin** (Synercid)
	Erythromycin (E-Mycin)	**Telithromycin** (Ketek)
	Fluconazole (Diflucan)	**Troleandomycin** (TAO)
	Itraconazole (Sporanox)	**Voriconazole** (Vfend)
	Ketoconazole (Nizoral)	

COMMENTS: Flibanserin is a CYP3A4 substrate, and antimicrobials that are CYP3A4 inhibitors may increase the risk of flibanserin toxicity.

CLASS 3: ASSESS RISK & TAKE ACTION IF NECESSARY
- *Consider Alternative*:
- Azole Antifungals: Itraconazole and ketoconazole are potent inhibitors of CYP3A4; fluconazole appears weaker, but in larger doses it also inhibits CYP3A4. **Terbinafine** (Lamisil) does not appear to affect CYP3A4, and would not be expected to interact with flibanserin.
  Macrolide Antibiotics: Unlike erythromycin, clarithromycin and troleandomycin, **azithromycin** (Zithromax) and **dirithromycin*** do not appear to inhibit CYP3A4. (*not available in US)
  Telithromycin: The use of **azithromycin** (Zithromax) or a quinolone antibiotic other than ciprofloxacin should be considered.
- *Monitor*: If flibanserin is used with CYP3A4 inhibitors, monitor for evidence of flibanserin toxicity such as hypotension, fainting, and CNS depression. Reduce flibanserin dose as needed.

OBJECT DRUGS	PRECIPITANT DRUGS
Flibanserin (Addyi)	**Calcium Channel Blockers:**
	Diltiazem (Cardizem)
	Verapamil (Isoptin)

COMMENTS: Flibanserin is a CYP3A4 substrate, and CYP3A4 inhibitors such as diltiazem or verapamil may increase the risk of flibanserin toxicity.

CLASS 3: ASSESS RISK & TAKE ACTION IF NECESSARY
- *Consider Alternative*: Calcium channel blockers other than diltiazem and verapamil are unlikely to inhibit the metabolism of flibanserin.
- *Monitor*: If flibanserin is used with CYP3A4 inhibitors, monitor for evidence of flibanserin toxicity such as hypotension, fainting, and CNS depression. Reduce flibanserin dose as needed.

OBJECT DRUGS	PRECIPITANT DRUGS	
Flibanserin (Addyi)	**Enzyme Inhibitors:**	
	Amiodarone (Cordarone)	**Delavirdine** (Rescriptor)
	Amprenavir (Agenerase)	**Dronedarone** (Multaq)
	Aprepitant (Emend)	**Grapefruit**
	Atazanavir (Reyataz)	**Indinavir** (Crixivan)
	Boceprevir (Victrelis)	**Lomitapide** (Juxtapid)
	Ceritinib (Zykadia)	**Mifepristone** (Korlym)
	Cimetidine (Tagamet)	**Nelfinavir** (Viracept)
	Cobicistat (Stribild)	**Ritonavir** (Norvir)
	Conivaptan (Vaprisol)	**Saquinavir** (Invirase)
	Cyclosporine (Neoral)	**Telaprevir** (Incivek)
	Darunavir (Prezista)	

COMMENTS: Flibanserin is a CYP3A4 substrate, and CYP3A4 inhibitors may increase the risk of flibanserin toxicity.

CLASS 3: ASSESS RISK & TAKE ACTION IF NECESSARY
- *Consider Alternative*:
  Cimetidine: **Famotidine** (Pepcid), **nizatidine** (Axid), and **ranitidine** (Zantac) have minimal effects on drug metabolism.
  Grapefruit: Orange juice does not appear to inhibit CYP3A4.
- *Monitor*: If flibanserin is used with CYP3A4 inhibitors, monitor for evidence of flibanserin toxicity such as hypotension, fainting, and CNS depression. Reduce flibanserin dose as needed.

OBJECT DRUGS	PRECIPITANT DRUGS	
Flibanserin (Addyi)	**Enzyme Inducers:**	
	Barbiturates	**Phenytoin** (Dilantin)
	Bosentan (Tracleer)	**Primidone** (Mysoline)
	Carbamazepine (Tegretol)	**Rifabutin** (Mycobutin)
	Dabrafenib (Tafinlar)	**Rifampin** (Rifadin)
	Dexamethasone (Decadron)	**Rifapentine** (Priftin)
	Efavirenz (Sustiva)	**St. John's wort**
	Lumacaftor (Orkambi)	
	Oxcarbazepine (Trileptal)	

COMMENTS: Flibanserin is metabolized by CYP3A4, and enzyme inducers may substantially reduce serum flibanserin concentrations. The product information for flibanserin states that enzyme inducers should not be administered with flibanserin.

CLASS 2: USE ONLY IF BENEFIT FELT TO OUTWEIGH RISK
- *Use Alternative*: The product information states that strong CYP3A4 inducers (phenytoin, carbamazepine, rifampin, St. John's wort) are contraindicated with flibanserin, but it would be best to avoid any enzyme inducer if possible.
  Anticonvulsants: In patients on flibanserin it would be desirable to use anticonvulsants that are not enzyme inducers, but in many cases it may not be reasonable to change the patient's anticonvulsant regimen.
  HIV Medications. Since most antiviral medications are either inducers or inhibitors of CYP3A4, it may not be possible to avoid these interactions in most cases.
  St. John's wort: Given the questionable benefit of St. John's wort, it would be prudent to avoid giving it with flibanserin.

- *Circumvent/Minimize:* If flibanserin is used with enzyme inducers, it may be necessary to increase the flibanserin dose.
- *Monitor:* If flibanserin is used with CYP3A4 inducers, monitor for evidence of reduced daclatasvir effect.

OBJECT DRUGS	PRECIPITANT DRUGS
Deferasirox (Exjade)	**Absorption Inhibitors:**
	Aluminum Antacids
	Cholestyramine (Questran)
	Colesevelam (WelChol)
	Colestipol (Colestid)

COMMENTS: Theoretically, the absorption of deferasirox may be reduced by agents containing aluminum. Cholestyramine moderately reduces deferasirox absorption, and other bile acid sequestrants probably have a similar effect.

CLASS 3: ASSESS RISK & TAKE ACTION IF NECESSARY
- *Circumvent/Minimize:* If combined therapy is necessary, give the deferasirox at least 2 to 4 hours before or 6 hours after the absorption inhibitor to minimize the interaction.
- *Monitor:* Watch for reduced deferasirox efficacy in patients taking absorption inhibitors.

Effect of Other Antibiotics on Warfarin

Antibiotics that are not inhibitors of CYP2C9 have been noted to increase the response to warfarin. It is important to note that both infection and inflammation can alter warfarin metabolism by increasing the production of cytokines. Several cytokines have been noted to reduce the activity of CYP2C9, the enzyme primarily responsible for the metabolism of S-warfarin, as well as other enzymes important for warfarin metabolism. When one considers the effect of cytokines combined with possible reduced intake of vitamin K during acute illness and fever-induced increase in catabolism of clotting factors, it is not unexpected that patients requiring antibiotics may have increased warfarin effect. This change in warfarin response may occur at the same time as antibiotic administration, but be unrelated to the administration of the antibiotic. Also evidence suggests that patients on warfarin who receive anti-infective agents may have a higher risk of hospitalization for gastrointestinal bleeding.

Antibiotic	Effect on Warfarin
Cephalosporins (NMTT side chain)	Cephalosporins with an NMTT side chain such as **cefoperazone** (Cefobid), **cefamandole** (Mandol), **cefotetan** (Cefotan), and **moxalactam** (Moxam) have been associated with hypoprothrombinemia.
Macrolides and Ketolides	**Erythromycin** produces small increases in warfarin response in most people but occasionally marked increases occur. **Clarithromycin** (Biaxin) and **telithromycin** (Ketek), like erythromycin, have been reported to increase warfarin effect. Isolated cases of increased warfarin effect reported with **azithromycin** (Zithromax) and a retrospective study found a small increase in INRs following azithromycin.
Penicillins	Occasionally, IV **ticarcillin** (Ticar) and to a lesser extent **mezlocillin** (Mezlin) and **piperacillin** (Pipracil) produce coagulation disorders (prolonged bleeding or increased INR). Isolated cases of increased warfarin effect reported with various penicillins such as amoxicillin, high dose IV penicillin G; the clinical importance is not known.
Quinolones	Several cases of elevated INRs have occurred when **moxifloxacin** (Avelox) was added to warfarin therapy. Isolated cases of increased warfarin effect reported with other quinolones such as **ciprofloxacin** (Cipro), **levofloxacin** (Levaquin),), **nalidixic acid** (NegGram), **norfloxacin** (Noroxin), and **ofloxacin** (Floxin), but a causal relationship is not clear in most cases; most quinolones do not appear to affect warfarin pharmacokinetics or hypoprothrombinemia but it may occur occasionally.
Tetracyclines	Isolated cases of increased warfarin effect with various tetracyclines; clinical importance not established.

Drug Interactions with Drugs that Increase QTc Intervals

A variety of drugs can affect the electrical activity of cardiac muscle. Normal cardiac contraction requires a rapid depolarization of the muscle followed by a slower repolarization. Repolarization is primarily accomplished by potassium efflux from the cell. Drugs can delay repolarization and prolong the cardiac action potential by blocking this potassium efflux. The delayed repolarization can be seen on the ECG as a prolongation of the QTc interval. Delayed repolarization enables an inward flow of calcium and premature depolarization. Early afterdepolarizations can trigger arrhythmias including torsades de pointes.

Some antiarrhythmic drugs such as amiodarone, procainamide, quinidine, sotalol, and dofetilide prolong repolarization as part of their therapeutic action and do so at therapeutic plasma concentrations. The incidence of torsades de pointes with these drugs has been noted to be <5 per 100 patients. Other drugs, not classified as antiarrhythmic agents, e.g., phenothiazines, tricyclic antidepressants, and some antibiotics, also slow repolarization by affecting potassium efflux. At plasma concentrations above usual therapeutic levels, these drugs may also produce arrhythmias. The risk of torsades de pointes is much less likely with these agents; perhaps 1 per 100,000 patients, although the exact incidence is not known.

Normal QTc duration is less than 440ms while QTc durations exceeding 500ms are more frequently associated with arrhythmias. QTc may vary by as much as 50 - 75ms over a 24 hour period in normal individuals. There is no agreement on the degree of QTc prolongation that is considered safe. Some believe no amount of increase is safe while others are not concerned with increases <35ms provided normal limits are not exceeded. Several factors including hypokalemia, hypomagnesemia, bradycardia, hypertrophy, heart failure, and female gender may predispose patients to increased clinical risk from prolonged QTc intervals. Although a prolonged QTc does not often lead to arrhythmias, patients with large QTc prolongations (e.g., > 60ms above baseline or those exceeding 500ms) may be at the greatest risk to develop arrhythmias including torsades de pointes.

We have classified the management of various combinations of QTc prolongating drugs (page 106) based on their risk and mechanism of the potential interaction. The table on page 107 categorizes some drugs that have been noted to increase the QTc interval. They are grouped based on their ability to alter the QTc at therapeutic or elevated plasma concentrations. Data are very limited regarding the ability of these drugs to induce arrhythmias when used alone or in combination. However, caution should be used when combinations of these agents are prescribed, particularly if the combination results in a pharmacokinetic interaction. Refer to the table on page 108 to identify combinations with potential pharmacokinetic interactions and those combinations that are limited to pharmacodynamic interactions and thus less likely to produce an arrhythmia. Consider substituting related drugs that do not affect the QTc interval as alternatives to one of the potentially interacting drugs. For example, SSRI antidepressants that do not inhibit CYP450 enzymes could be used in place of tricyclic antidepressants, or a quinolone without potential cardiac effects could be substituted for a quinolone reported to prolong the QTc interval.

Management Classes for Prolonged QTc Interval Drug Interactions
(For Use With Drug Charts on Next Page)

Management Class 1: Avoid Combination.

a. Any two drugs from Column I. (e.g., Dofetilide + Quinidine)

b. A drug from Column I plus a drug from Column II that also have a pharmacokinetic interaction. (e.g., Quinidine + Clarithromycin)

Management Class 2: Use only if Benefit Felt to Outweigh Risk.

a. A drug from Column I plus a drug from Column II that *do not* have a pharmacokinetic interaction (pharmacodynamic interaction only). (e.g., Procainamide + Haloperidol)

b. Any two drugs from Column II that *also* have a pharmacokinetic interaction. (e.g., Cisapride + Erythromycin)

c. Any drug from Column I plus a drug that produces a pharmacokinetic interaction. (e.g., Quinidine + Ketoconazole)

Management Class 3: Assess risk and take action if necessary.

a. Any two drugs from Column II that *do not* have a pharmacokinetic interaction (pharmacodynamic interaction only). (e.g., Clozapine + Ziprasidone)

b. A drug from Column II plus a drug that inhibits its metabolism. (e.g., Amitriptyline + Diphenhydramine)

Note: Class 2 and 3 drug combinations should be administered only with ECG monitoring for potential changes in QTc interval; when appropriate, also monitor the plasma concentration of the antiarrhythmic drug.

Drugs Reported to Prolong the QTc Interval[a]

Column I Drugs that prolong the QTc interval at therapeutic concentrations.	Column II Drugs that may produce clinically relevant prolongation of the QTc interval at elevated concentrations.
Amiodarone (Cordarone)	Amitriptyline (Elavil)[b]
Arsenic trioxide (Trisenox)	Chloroquine (Aralen)
Bedaquiline (Sirturo)	Chlorpromazine (Thorazine)
Bepridil Vascor)	Cisapride (Propulsid)
Ceritinib (Zykadia)	Clarithromycin (Biaxin)
Disopyramide (Norpace)	Clomipramine (Anafranil)[b]
Dofetilide (Tikosyn)	Clozapine (Clozaril)
Dronedarone (Multaq)	Crizotinib (Xalkori)
Flecainide (Tambocor)	Desipramine (Norpramin)
Halofantrine (Halfan)	Dolasetron (Anzemet)
Ibutilide (Covert)	Droperidol (Inapsine)
Lapatinib (Tykerb)	Erythromycin (E-Mycin)
Lumefantrine (Coartem)	Gatifloxacin (Tequin)
Mesoridazine (Serentil)	Haloperidol (Haldol)
Pimozide (Orap)	Iloperidone (Fanapt)
Procainamide (Procanbid)	Levomethadyl (Orlaam)
N-acetylprocainamide	Mefloquine (Lariam)
Quinidine (Quinidex)	Methadone (Dolophine)
Sotalol (Betapace)	Moxifloxacin (Avelox)
Thioridazine (Mellaril)	Nilotinib (Tasigna)
Vandetanib (Caprelsa)	Ondansetron (Zofran)
	Ranolazine (Ranexa)
	Sumatriptan (Imitrex)
	Ziprasidone (Geodon)
	Zolmitriptan (Zomig)

a. Note that the lists are not exhaustive, nor should a drug's listing in a specific column be considered absolute. As additional data become available, drug listings are subject to change. Some drugs have profound effects on QTc while others produce only minor changes, particularly in the absence of predisposing factors.
b. Widens the QRS interval.

Drugs Reported to Prolong QTc Intervals:
Known Substrates and Inhibitors of CYP2D6 and CYP3A4

CYP Enzyme	Substrates	Inhibitors[c]
CYP2D6	Amitriptyline[a] Chlorpromazine Clomipramine[a] Desipramine Flecainide (Tambocor) Haloperidol Mesoridazine (Serentil) Propafenone Thioridazine	Amiodarone Dronedarone Haloperidol Lumefantrine Quinidine Thioridazine
CYP3A4	Amiodarone Amitriptyline Bedaquiline Bepridil Ceritinib (Zykadia) Cisapride Clomipramine Crizotinib Disopyramide Dofetilide[b] Dronedarone Droperidol Halofantrine (Halfan) Lapatinib Levomethadyl Lumefantrine Nilotinib Ondansetron Pimozide Quinidine Ranolazine Ziprasidone[d]	Amiodarone Clarithromycin Crizotinib Dronedarone Erythromycin Lapatinib

a. CYP2D6 is the primary pathway
b. Dofetilide has about 70% renal elimination
c. Other drugs that inhibit CYP2D6 or CYP3A4 may also interact. See the Table Cytochrome P450 Enzymes and Transporters for more potential inhibitors of the substrates listed above.
d. Ziprasidone is about 33% metabolized by CYP3A4; aldehyde oxidase metabolizes most of the remainder.

Genetic Polymorphisms of Cytochrome P450 Enzymes

The pharmacogenetics of drug-metabolizing enzymes contributes to the variability observed between patients receiving the same two interacting drugs at the same doses. Differences in the genetic makeup of enzymes (genotype) can lead to altered patient responses including toxicity or lack of efficacy (phenotype). The table below lists common CYP450 enzymes known to have different phenotypes. Differing phenotypes result in patients that are often referred to as extensive or poor metabolizers of drugs that are substrates for a specific cytochrome P450 enzyme. Poor metabolizers (PMs) will accumulate more of the parent drug. However, since their ability to metabolize the drug is limited, they are protected from other drugs that may inhibit the enzyme. Extensive metabolizers (EMs), usually the most common phenotype, will have greater (normal) enzyme activity and lower concentrations of the parent drug. EMs often demonstrate large reductions in the metabolism of object drugs when an inhibitor is coadministered and are at greater risk of developing an adverse outcome from a drug interaction than PMs. Ultra rapid metabolizers (UMs) have extra functional copies of the gene and therefore have very rapid substrate metabolism. These UMs may be the most affected by the concurrent administration of an inhibitor. Polymorphisms are clinically most important for drugs with a narrow therapeutic range and when the polymorphic pathway is responsible for a major portion of the drug's metabolism.

Enzyme	Frequency of phenotype	Examples of drugs affected
CYP2C9	PM 6-10% Caucasians PM 8% Asian PM 10-14% African Americans	Glyburide, Glipizide, Warfarin, Phenytoin
CYP2C19	PM 3-5% Caucasians PM 12-23% Asians PM 10-20% African Americans UM 5% Caucasians	Diazepam, Omeprazole, Pantoprazole
CYP2D6	PM 6-14% Caucasians PM 3-6% Hispanic PM 2-5% African Americans PM 5-10% Asians[a] UM 1-4% Caucasians[b]	Codeine, Imipramine, Propafenone, Metoprolol
CYP2B6	PM 15-27% Caucasians PM 10 – 20% Asian PM 33-50% African Americans	Bupropion, Efavirenz, Methadone
CYP3A4	Under Study	Numerous (about half of all drugs are metabolized by CYP3A4/5)
CYP3A5	PM 90-95% Caucasians PM 70-75% Asian PM 30-35% African Americans	Numerous (about half of all drugs are metabolized by CYP3A4/5)

a. Roughly half of Asians are "Intermediate Metabolizers" of CYP2D6, meaning that they have CYP2D6 activity that is in between "Poor Metabolizers" and "Rapid Metabolizers."

b. Approximate prevalence of "Ultra rapid" CYP2D6 metabolizers: Finns and Danes 1%; North Americans (white) 4%; Greeks 10%; Portuguese 10%; Saudis 20%; Ethiopians 30%. Such people may have low concentrations of CYP2D6 substrates, and may also develop morphine toxicity when given the pro-drug codeine.

Drug Interactions with Herbal Products

There has been increasing attention to the interactions of medications with herbal products, and some herbal drug interactions are relatively well documented. For example, ephedrine is an indirect-acting sympathomimetic that may result in acute hypertension when combined with MAO inhibitors. Kava and valerian have well-documented sedative properties, and may have additive effects with other CNS depressant drugs. St. John's wort is an inducer of CYP3A4, and probably also induces CYP2C9 and P-glycoprotein. It appears to interact with a variety of drugs that are substrates for these isozymes and transporters.

Other purported drug interactions of herbal products are not as well documented, and a causal relationship has not been established. For example the purported ability of many herbal products to increase the risk of bleeding in patients receiving warfarin is based primarily on isolated case reports and in vitro/animal studies. Several herbal products reportedly inhibit platelet function, thereby increasing the risk of bleeding in patients on oral anticoagulants, but there is very little supporting clinical evidence. Many other suspected herbal-drug interactions are based on similarly inadequate clinical information.

Moreover, prevention of adverse drug-herbal interactions is hampered by several other factors. Herbal medications are usually not standardized, so different herbal brands may interact differently with other medications due to different amounts of active ingredient or additional ingredients not on the label (and in some cases no active ingredients at all). Moreover, different lots of the same brand may vary substantially as to content as well. Herbal medications are often absent from computerized drug interaction screening systems, so it is important to educate patients to keep their health professionals informed of all alternative medications. **Note**: Some herbal drug interactions are included in the preceding monographs, and can be found by consulting the index.

Object Drugs	Precipitant Drugs

Aliskiren (Tekturna) — Grapefruit
Grapefruit juice (200 mL TID X 5 days) substantially reduced aliskiren plasma concentrations, probably by inhibition of OATP2B1. The magnitude of the effect suggests that aliskiren effect is likely to be reduced.

Alprazolam (Xanax) — St. John's wort
St. John's wort substantially reduces alprazolam plasma concentrations, and would be expected to reduce alprazolam response. Other benzodiazepines that are CYP3A4 substrates (e.g., midazolam, triazolam) may be similarly affected.

Amygdalin — Vitamin C
A cancer patient on vitamin C 4800 mg/day developed cyanide toxicity with seizures and lactic acidosis soon after taking one dose of amygdalin, possibly through increased conversion of amygdalin to cyanide. Although more data are needed, the severity of the reaction suggests that patients taking amygdalin avoid high dose vitamin C.

Antidepressants:
(norepinephrine uptake inhibitors)   Yohimbine
Amitriptyline (Elavil)
Amoxapine (Asendin)
Clomipramine (Anafranil)
Desipramine (Norpramin)
Desvenlafaxine (Pristiq)
Doxepin (Sinequan)
Duloxetine (Cymbalta)
Imipramine (Tofranil)
Levomilnacipran (Fetzima)
Milnacipran (Savella)
Mirtazapine (Remeron)
Nortriptyline (Aventyl)
Protriptyline (Vivactil)
Trimipramine (Surmontil)
Venlafaxine (Effexor)

Yohimbine increases synaptic norepinephrine release through inhibition of alpha-2 adrenergic receptors, and many antidepressants inhibit norepinephrine reuptake. Concurrent administration of yohimbine with the norepinephrine uptake inhibitor atomoxetine has been shown to increase blood pressure, and isolated case reports indicate that combining yohimbine with antidepressant norepinephrine inhibitors such as clomipramine may increase blood pressure. Monitor blood pressure response.

Atomoxetine (Strattera)   **Yohimbine**

Yohimbine increases synaptic norepinephrine release through inhibition of alpha-2 adrenergic receptors, and atomoxetine inhibits norepinephrine reuptake. Concurrent administration of yohimbine with atomoxetine has been shown to increase blood pressure, which has been used intentionally in patients with peripheral autonomic failure. Monitor blood pressure in patients receiving the combination.

Bupropion (Wellbutrin)   **St. John's wort**

St. John's wort modestly reduced bupropion plasma concentrations in healthy subjects, and it is possible that some patients may develop decreased bupropion efficacy if St. John's wort is used concurrently. A case of orofacial dystonia occurred in a patient taking bupropion and St. John's wort, but a causal relationship was not established.

Buspirone (BuSpar)   **St. John's wort**

Isolated cases have been reported of possible serotonin syndrome or hypomania following concurrent use of buspirone and St. John's wort, but a causal relationship was not established.

Calcium-channel Blockers   **St. John's wort**

See monograph on page 32.

Carbamazepine   **Piperine**

Piperine has been shown to modestly increase carbamazepine plasma concentrations in patients receiving carbamazepine for epilepsy. The mechanism for this effect is not established. The effect was not large, but it would be prudent to monitor for carbamazepine toxicity if piperine is used concurrently.

Carbamazepine   **Resveratrol**

Resveratrol moderately increased carbamazepine plasma concentrations in healthy subjects; more data are needed to establish the clinical importance of this interaction.

CNS Depressants: **Kava**
Alcohol
Barbiturates
Benzodiazepines
Opiates

Kava is a central nervous system depressant, and may have additive depressant effects with other CNS depressants. Monitor patient for evidence of excessive CNS depression.

111

CNS Depressants:
Alcohol
Barbiturates
Benzodiazepines
Opiates   **Valerian**

Valerain is a central nervous system depressant, and may have additive depressant effects with other CNS depressants. Monitor patient for evidence of excessive CNS depression.

Contraceptives, Oral   **St. John's wort**
See monograph on page 42.

Daclatasvir (Daklinza)   **St. John's wort**
Daclatasvir is a CYP3A4 substrate and St. John's wort is likely to substantially reduce daclatasvir plasma concentrations. Avoid concurrent use if possible.

Dextromethorphan   **Berberine (Goldenseal)**
Berberine markedly increases dextromethorphan plasma concentrations, probably through inhibition of CYP2D6. Monitor for adverse effects of dextromethorphan, including nervousness, confusion, nausea and tremors.

Digoxin (Lanoxin)   **Ginseng**
A case of increased digoxin serum concentrations following Siberian ginseng has been reported, possibly due to interference with digoxin assay. The clinical importance of this purported interaction is not established, but one should monitor for altered digoxin concentrations and response when any herbal product is added (many herbal products reportedly contain digoxin-like substances).

Digoxin   **Sennosides (Senna)**
Evidence from a nested case-control study suggested that use of senna laxatives is associated with an increased risk of hospitalization for digoxin toxicity. Theoretically, laxative-induced hypokalemia could increase digoxin toxicity, but more data are needed to establish the clinical importance of this interaction.

Digoxin (Lanoxin)   **St. John's wort**
Pharmacokinetic study in healthy subjects suggest that St. John's wort may modestly reduce digoxin serum concentrations, probably due to St. John's wort-induced increase in P-glycoprotein activity. The extent to which this interaction would result in reduced digoxin efficacy is not known. Monitor patients for reduced digoxin response and digoxin serum concentrations.

Erlotinib (Tarceva)   **St. John's wort**
See monograph on page 61.

Erythromycin   **St. John's wort**
In healthy subjects, St. John's wort produced a 1.4-fold increase in erythromycin demethylation probably through increased CYP3A4 activity. The magnitude of this effect suggests that St. John's wort may reduce erythromycin efficacy in some patients. Clarithromycin and azithromycin are also metabolized by CYP3A4 and may interact similarly with St. John's wort.

Felodipine (Plendil)   **Peppermint Oil**
Peppermint oil moderately increased felodipine plasma concentrations, but the clinical importance of this interaction is not established.

Fexofenadine (Allegra)   **St. John's wort**
St. John's wort can substantially reduce the plasma concentration of fexofenadine. Avoid concurrent use.

Finasteride (Proscar)   **St. John's wort**
St. John's wort produced a 35% decrease in plasma finasteride concentrations in healthy subjects, probably through increased CYP3A4 activity. The magnitude of this effect suggests that St. John's wort may reduce finasteride efficacy in some patients. **Dutasteride** (Avodart) is also metabolized by CYP3A4 and may interact similarly with St. John's wort.

112

Glicazide*   **St. John's wort**

St. John's wort modestly reduced (35% decrease) plasma concentrations of glicazide in healthy subjects. Although the clinical importance of this effect requires further study, it is possible that St. John's wort could reduce glicazide efficacy in some patients.
* Not available in United States

Glipizide (Glucotrol)   **St. John's wort**

St. John's wort can reduce the plasma concentration of glipizide. St. John's wort should generally be avoided in patients taking glipizide.

Ibuprofen (Advil, Motrin)   **St. John's wort**

St. John's wort can reduce the plasma concentration of ibuprofen. St. John's wort should generally be avoided in patients taking ibuprofen.

Imatinib (Gleevec)   **St. John's wort**

See monograph on page 61.

Immunosuppressants: **Boldo**
Cyclosporine (Neoral)
Sirolimus (Rapamune)
Tacrolimus (Prograf)

Limited clinical evidence suggests that use of boldo may result in subtherapeutic tacrolimus concentrations. More data are needed to establish the clinical importance of this effect.

Immunosuppressants: **Echinacea**
Cyclosporine (Neoral)
Sirolimus (Rapamune)
Tacrolimus (Prograf)

Echinacea purportedly may reduce the efficacy of cyclosporine and other immunosuppressants. This is based on theoretical considerations, however, and the clinical importance of this purported interaction is unknown.

Immunosuppressants: **St. John's wort**
Cyclosporine (Neoral)
Sirolimus (Rapamune)
Tacrolimus (Prograf)

See monograph on page xx.

Immunosuppressants: **Zinc**
Cyclosporine (Neoral)
Sirolimus (Rapamune)
Tacrolimus (Prograf)

Zinc, acting as an "immunostimulant", purportedly may reduce the efficacy of cyclosporine and other immunosuppressants. This is based on theoretical considerations, however, and the clinical importance of this purported interaction is unknown.

Indinavir (Crixivan)   **St. John's wort**

See monograph on page 24.

Irinotecan (Camptosar)   **St. John's wort**

St. John's wort can substantially reduce irinotecan plasma concentrations; St. John's wort should generally be avoided in patients on irinotecan.

Ivabradine (Corlanor)   **St. John's wort**

St. John's wort substantially reduced ivabradine plasma concentrations in healthy subjects, probably through increased CYP3A4 activity. It is possible that some patients may develop decreased ivabradine efficacy if St. John's wort is used concurrently.

Ledipasvir/sofosbuvir (Harvoni)   **St. John's wort**

Both ledipasvir and sofosbuvir are substrates for P-glycoprotein, and St. John's wort is likely to reduce their plasma concentrations by increasing P-glycoprotein activity.

Levodopa   **Kava**

A patient with Parkinson's disease treated with levodopa had increased "off" periods during kava use. Confirmation is needed, but monitor for altered efficacy of antiparkinson drugs if kava is used.

Loperamide (Imodium) St. John's wort
A patient on concurrent loperamide, St. John's wort and valerian developed delirium, but a causal relationship was not established.

Losartan (Cozaar) Berberine (Goldenseal)
Berberine substantially decreases the conversion of losartan to its active metabolite probably through inhibition of CYP2C9. Theoretically, this should result in reduced losartan effects. Although the clinical importance of this interaction is not established, it would be prudent to monitor losartan effect if berberine is started or stopped.

MAO Inhibitors Ephedrine
Severe hypertensive reactions are likely, and the combination is contraindicated. See monograph on page 68.

MAO Inhibitors Ginseng
The use of ginseng has been associated with isolated cases of toxicity (e.g., headache, insomnia, irritability, and tremor) in patients receiving phenelzine (Nardil), but a causal relationship was not established. Although the potential interaction is poorly documented, given the lack of evidence of ginseng efficacy, the combination would best be avoided. If the combination is used the patient should be carefully monitored for adverse effects.

Melatonin Fluvoxamine (Luvox)
Based on a pharmacokinetic study in healthy subjects, fluvoxamine may produce a marked increase in melatonin serum concentrations. Although the clinical importance of this effect is not established, one should watch for evidence of excessive melatonin effect if the combination is used.

Mephenytoin St. John's wort
In a pharmacokinetic study in healthy subjects, St. John's wort significantly reduced mephenytoin plasma concentrations through increased CYP2C19 activity. Reduced mephenytoin effect should be expected.

Midazolam (Versed) Berberine (Goldenseal)
Berberine appears to moderately increase midazolam plasma concentrations (about 40%) following oral midazolam, probably through inhibition of CYP3A4. Non-oral routes of midazolam administration are not likely to be affected as much. Monitor for enhanced midazolam response.

Midazolam (Versed) Echinacea
In healthy subjects echinacea increased oral midazolam plasma concentrations and decreased intravenous midazolam plasma concentrations. But the evidence is somewhat conflicting, and the clinical importance of these interactions is not established.

Midazolam (Versed) Ginkgo
Ginkgo appears to moderately reduce midazolam plasma concentrations (about 34%) following oral midazolam, probably by increasing CYP3A4 activity. Non-oral routes of midazolam administration are not likely to be affected as much. Monitor for reduced midazolam response.

Midazolam (Versed) St. John's wort
Several studies have shown that St. John's wort reduces plasma concentrations of midazolam. The effect is likely to be greater with oral than with parenteral midazolam administration.

Methotrexate Glutamine
A case of severe methotrexate toxicity during use of glutamine has been reported in a 14-year-old boy with lymphoma. More study is needed to establish the clinical importance of this potential interaction, but patients on the combination should be carefully monitored for methotrexate toxicity.

Nevirapine (Viramune) St. John's wort
In five HIV positive patients, the use of St. John's wort was associated with reduced nevirapine plasma concentrations compared with the same patients without St. John's wort. A database of 176 patients on nevirapine also suggested reduced nevirapine plasma concentrations with St. John's wort. Patients on nevirapine should probably avoid taking St. John's wort.

Nifedipine (Procardia)   **Melatonin**

Hypertensive patients stabilized on nifedipine developed increased blood pressure after the use of melatonin. The clinical importance of this effect is not established.

NSAIDs   **Ginkgo**

Ginkgo and NSAIDS purportedly may display additive inhibitory effects on platelet function, but the clinical importance of this effect is unknown.

Omeprazole (Prilosec)   **St. John's wort**

In healthy subjects St. John's wort reduced omeprazole plasma concentrations by about 40%. Although the clinical importance of this effect is not established, one should be alert for reduced omeprazole effect.

Oxycodone (Percocet)   **St. John's wort**

See monograph on page 76.

Phenytoin (Dilantin)   **Ginkgo**

Fatal seizures occurred in an epileptic man on phenytoin and valproic acid who took ginkgo (and several other herbal medicines) concurrently. There is some clinical evidence to suggest that ginkgo may increase CYP2C19 activity, so it is possible that the ginkgo reduced phenytoin (and possibly valproic acid) plasma concentrations. More evidence is needed to establish a causal relationship.

Phenytoin (Dilantin)   **Piperine**

Piperine has been shown to moderately increase phenytoin plasma concentrations in both healthy subjects and in patients receiving phenytoin for epilepsy. The mechanism for this effect is not established. More data are needed to establish the clinical importance of this interaction, but it would be prudent to monitor for phenytoin toxicity if piperine is used concurrently.

Phenytoin (Dilantin)   **St. John's wort**

St. John's wort substantially increased the CYP2C19 metabolism of mephenytoin in healthy subjects, and other evidence suggests that St. John's wort increases CYP2C9 activity. Since CYP2C19 and CYP2C9 are the isozymes primarily responsible for the metabolism of phenytoin, one would expect reduced phenytoin efficacy in at least some patients if St. John's wort is used concurrently.

Quazepam (Doral)   **St. John's wort**

St. John's wort modestly reduced zolpidem plasma concentrations (26%) in healthy subjects, probably through induction of CYP3A4. It is possible that some patients may develop decreased quazepam efficacy if St. John's wort is used concurrently. Most other benzodiazepines (as well as zaleplon and zopiclone) are metabolized by CYP3A4 and may interact similarly with St. John's wort.

Raltegravir (Isentress)   **Ginkgo**

Ginkgo (240 mg/day for 15 days) modestly increased plasma concentrations of raltegravir in healthy subjects, but the clinical importance of the interaction is probably minimal in most patients.

Risperidone (Risperdal)   **Ginkgo**

A case of priapism has been reported in a man taking risperidone and ginkgo, but a causal relationship was not established.

Rosuvastatin (Crestor)   **Baicalin**

Baicalin may reduce rosuvastatin plasma concentrations, probably by inducing OATP. Baicalin is found in several Chinese herbal products.

Saquinavir (Invirase)   **Garlic**

Garlic capsules substantially reduced saquinavir serum concentrations in healthy subjects. Although confirmation is needed, it would be prudent to monitor for reduced saquinavir effect if garlic is used concurrently. In another study, garlic did not affect ritonavir pharmacokinetics in healthy subjects.

Selective Serotonin Reuptake   **St. John's wort**
Inhibitors (SSRIs)

St. John's wort has reportedly produced serotonin syndrome when given to patients receiving SSRIs. The symptoms reported, however, have not been the classic findings of serotonin syndrome. Although the evidence for an interaction is minimal it would be prudent to watch for evidence of serotonin syndrome. Serotonin syndrome can result in neurotoxicity (myoclonus, tremors, rigidity, incoordination, hyperreflexia, seizures, coma), psychiatric symptoms (agitation, confusion, hypomania, restlessness), and autonomic dysfunction (fever, sweating, tachycardia, hypertension).

Talinolol   Ginkgo
Ginkgo may modestly increase talinolol plasma concentrations, but the clinical importance of the interaction is not established.

Theophylline   St. John's wort
A case of possible St. John's wort-induced reduction in plasma theophylline concentrations has been reported, but this was not confirmed by a study of the interaction in healthy subjects. The latter finding is consistent with several trials finding little or no effect of St. John's wort on caffeine pharmacokinetics, a substance whose metabolism is similar to that of theophylline.

Valproic Acid   Chitosan
Two patients receiving valproic acid for epilepsy developed seizures after starting chitosan for weight loss. Both cases rated a "probable" causal relationship based on the Drug Interaction Probability Scale (DIPS). Pending additional data on this interaction, it would be prudent to avoid chitosan in people taking valproic acid.

Verapamil (Calan)   St. John's wort
See monograph on page 32.

Voriconazole (Vfend)   St. John's wort
St. John's wort reduced the concentration of voriconazole by over 50%. Avoid concurrent use.

Warfarin (Coumadin)   Boldo-Fenugreek
A patient stabilized on warfarin developed an increased INR after starting a herbal product containing boldo-fenugreek. A positive dechallenge and rechallenge suggests a causal relationship. If boldo-fenugreek is used with warfarin, monitor for bleeding and changes in INR.

Warfarin (Coumadin)   Chitosan
Chitosan was associated with an increased INR on two occasions in a patient on chronic warfarin therapy. The effect appeared causal in this patient, but more study is needed. Pending additional data on this interaction, it would be prudent to avoid chitosan in people taking warfarin or other coumarin anticoagulants.

Warfarin (Coumadin)   Coenzyme Q10
Several cases have been reported of reduced hypoprothrombinemic response in patients receiving warfarin who received coenzyme Q10 concomitantly. Although a causal relationship was not established, the combination would be best avoided; if it is used the patient should be carefully monitored for changes in INR.

Warfarin (Coumadin)   Cranberry
Cranberry juice or sauce has been implicated in several cases of marked INR increases in patients on warfarin; at least two cases were fatal. Nonetheless, several controlled studies have found little or no effect of cranberry juice on either warfarin pharmacokinetics or anticoagulant response.

Warfarin (Coumadin)   Danshen
Danshen has been associated with several cases of increased hypoprothrombinemic response and bleeding in patients receiving warfarin. Although a causal relationship has not been conclusively established, the combination would be best avoided. If the combination is used, the patient should be carefully monitored for increased INR and bleeding.

Warfarin (Coumadin)   Dong Quai
Dong quai has been associated with isolated cases of increased hypoprothrombinemic response in patients on warfarin. Dong quai purportedly also inhibits platelet function. Although the clinical importance of this effect is unknown, as with any drug added to warfarin, the patient should be monitored for evidence of bleeding and changes in INR.

Warfarin (Coumadin)   Feverfew

Feverfew purportedly may increase the risk of bleeding in patients on warfarin due to inhibition of platelet function, but the clinical importance of this effect is unknown. As with any drug added to warfarin, the patient should be monitored for evidence of bleeding and changes in INR.

Warfarin (Coumadin)　　　　Garlic
Garlic supplements purportedly increase the risk of bleeding due to inhibition of platelet function, but the clinical importance of this effect is questionable. In a crossover study of healthy subjects, garlic did not affect the INR response to warfarin. Another study also failed to find an interaction between garlic and warfarin. Although most evidence suggests that garlic does not interact with warfarin, patients should still be monitored for evidence of bleeding and changes in INR if garlic products are used. There is no evidence that garlic in food affects the bleeding risk in patients on warfarin.

Warfarin (Coumadin)　　　　Ginger
Ginger purportedly may increase the risk of bleeding due to inhibition of platelet function, but the clinical importance of this effect is unknown. Study in healthy subjects suggests that ginger does not affect warfarin pharmacokinetics. If the combination is used, patients should be monitored for evidence of bleeding and changes in INR.

Warfarin (Coumadin)　　　　Ginkgo
Ginkgo has been associated with isolated cases of severe bleeding in patients receiving warfarin or aspirin, but a causal relationship was not established. Some evidence suggests that ginkgo inhibits platelet function, an effect that would not be reflected in an increased INR. Nonetheless, most trials have failed to find an effect of ginkgo on platelets or blood coagulation. As with any drug added to warfarin therapy, one should be alert for increased bleeding, but special precautions do not appear necessary at this time.

Warfarin (Coumadin)　　　　Ginseng
Isolated case reports and study in healthy subjects suggest that ginseng can reduce the effect of warfarin. Most studies, however, suggest that ginseng has no effect on platelets or warfarin response. Nonetheless, given the lack of evidence of ginseng efficacy, the combination should generally be avoided. If the combination is used, patients should be monitored for altered INR.

Warfarin (Coumadin)　　　　Glucosamine
A number of case reports suggest that glucosamine can increase the effect of warfarin, but most of the cases have been spontaneous reports to adverse reaction database agencies. A causal relationship is not established. Pending additional information, monitored for altered INR if the combination is used.

Warfarin (Coumadin)　　　　Goji (lycium barbarum)
A patient on warfarin developed a markedly increased INR after drinking goji juice for several days. More data are needed to determine whether goji products affect warfarin response.

Warfarin (Coumadin)　　　　Green Tea
A patient on warfarin developed inhibition of the hypoprothrombinemic response after consuming large amounts of green tea daily (up to 1 gallon). Although a causal relationship was not established, until more information is available it would be prudent to advise patients on warfarin to avoid large amounts of green tea.

Warfarin (Coumadin)　　　　Menthol
Isolated cases of reduced warfarin response have been reported following use of menthol cough drops, but more study is needed to establish a causal relationship. Until more information is available, it would be prudent to monitor for reduced warfarin response if menthol cough drops are used.

Warfarin (Coumadin)　　　　Pomegranate
Isolated cases of increased warfarin response have been reported; more study is needed to establish the clinical importance.

Warfarin (Coumadin)　　　　Quilinggao
A patient stabilized on warfarin developed bleeding and an elevated INR after taking a Chinese herbal product containing quilinggao. Another brand of quilinggao later produced a similar effect. If quilinggao is used with warfarin, monitor for bleeding and changes in INR.

Warfarin (Coumadin)　　　　　　**St. John's wort**
See monograph on page 7.

Zolpidem (Ambien)　　　　　　**St. John's wort**
St. John's wort modestly reduced zolpidem plasma concentrations (30%) in healthy subjects, probably through induction of CYP3A4. It is possible that some patients may develop decreased zolpidem efficacy if St. John's wort is used concurrently. **Zaleplon, zopiclone,** and many benzodiazepines are also metabolized by CYP3A4 and may interact similarly with St. John's wort.

# INDEX
Underline = Class 1; *Italic* = Class 2; Roman = Class 3

120

122

123

125

126

127

128

129

131

133

137

138

Meperidine 77
Methadone 68
Methylene Blue 68
Nateglinide 16,17
Nelfinavir 77
NSAIDs 75
Olanzapine 21,37
Oxycodone 77
Paliperidone 21
Phenelzine 68
Phenytoin 78
Pimozide 81
Pioglitazone 17
Quinidine 4
Ramelteon 83
Ranolazine 84
Rasagiline 69
Repaglinide 17
Rifabutin 85
Rilpivirine 77
Risperidone 21
Ritonavir 77
Rosiglitazone 16
Saquinavir 77
Saxagliptin 17
Selegiline 69
Sildenafil 79
Simvastatin 55
Sirolimus 58
Sitagliptin 17
Sufentanil 77
Tacrolimus 58
Tadalafil 79
Tapentadol 78
Tasimelteon 83
Theophylline 89
Thiazide diuretics 90
Thioridazine 91
Tipranavir 77
Tizanidine 92
Tolbutamide 16
Tramadol 78
Tranylcypromine 68
Vardenafil 79
Vinblastine 95
Vincristine 95
Vinorelbine 95
Warfarin 9
Fosamprenavir. See
Amprenavir
Fosinopril. See ACE
Inhibitors
Fosphenytoin. See
Phenytoin
Frova. See Frovatriptan
Frovatriptan
Ergot Alkaloids 52
Fulvicin. See Griseofulvin
Furazolidone. See MAO
Inhibitors, Nonselective
Furoxone. See MAO
Inhibitors, Nonselective
Furosemide
Cholestyramine 48
Colestipol 48
Lithium 64

-G-
Galantamine
Acebutolol 39
Amitriptyline 37
Amoxapine 37
Atenolol 39
Atropine 38
Azatadine 37
Azelastine 37
Belladonna 38
Benztropine 38
Betaxolol 39
Biperiden 38
Bisoprolol 39
Brompheniramine 37
Carteolol 39
Carvedilol 39
Ceritinib 39
Chlorpheniramine 37
Chlorpromazine 38
Clemastine 37
Clidinium 38
Clomipramine 37
Clozapine 38
Cyclizine 37
Cyclobenzaprine 40
Cyproheptadine 37
Darifenacin 38
Desipramine 37
Dexchlorpheniramine 37
Dicyclomine 38
Digoxin 39
Dimenhydrinate 37
Doxepin 37
Esmolol 39
Fesoterodine 38
Flavoxate 38
Glycopyrrolate 38
Hydroxyzine 37
Hyoscyamine 38
Imipramine 37
Labetalol 39
Levobunolol 39
Meclizine 37
Methocarbamol 40
Methscopolamine 38
Metoprolol 39
Nadolol 39
Nebivolol 39
Nortriptyline 37
Olanzapine 38
Orphenadrine 40
Oxybutynin 38
Penbutolol 39
Pindolol 39
Prochlorperazine 37
Procyclidine 38
Promethazine 37
Propantheline 38
Propranolol 39
Protriptyline 37
Quetiapine 38
Scopolamine 37
Solifenacin 39
Sotalol 39
Thioridazine 38
Timolol 39

Tolterodine 38
Trifluoperazine 38
Trihexyphenidyl 38
Trimipramine 37
Triprolidine 37
Trospium 38
Garlic. See Herbal
Interaction Chart
Gaviscon. See Antacids
Gefitinib. See Kinase
inhibitors
Gelusil. See Antacids
Gemfibrozil
Atorvastatin 54
Lovastatin 54
Pitavastatin 54
Repaglinide 18
Rosuvastatin 54
Simvastatin 54
Warfarin 10
Gemifloxacin
Antacids 83
Calcium Polycarbophil 83
Corticosteroids 46
Didanosine 83
Iron 83
Sucralfate 83
Zinc 83
Geodon. See Ziprasidone
Ginger. See Herbal
Interaction Chart
Ginkgo. See Herbal
Interaction Chart
Ginseng. See Herbal
Interaction Chart
Gleevec. See Imatinib
Glimepiride
Amiodarone 16
Beta-blockers 15
Capecitabine 16
Ceritinib 16
Co-trimoxazole 16
Delavirdine 16
Efavirenz 16
Etravirine 16
Fluconazole 15
Fluoxetine 16
Fluorouracil 16
Fluvastatin 16
Fluvoxamine 16
Metronidazole 16
Miconazole 15
Sulfinpyrazone 16
Voriconazole 15
Glipizide. See Herbal
Interaction Chart
Amiodarone 16
Beta-blockers 15
Capecitabine 16
Ceritinib 16
Co-trimoxazole 16
Delavirdine 16
Efavirenz 16
Etravirine 16
Fluconazole 15
Fluoxetine 16
Fluorouracil 16

Fluvastatin 16
Fluvoxamine 16
Gastric Alkalinizers 18
Metronidazole 16
Miconazole 15
Sulfinpyrazone 16
Voriconazole 15
Glucophage. See
Metformin
Glucosamine.. See Herbal
Interaction Chart
Glucotrol. See Glipizide
Glucovance. See Glyburide
and Metformin
Glutamine. See Herbal
Interaction Chart
Glyburide
Amiodarone 16
Beta-blockers 15
Capecitabine 16
Ceritinib 16
Delavirdine 16
Efavirenz 16
Etravirine 16
Fluconazole 15
Fluoxetine 16
Fluorouracil 16
Fluvastatin 16
Fluvoxamine 16
Gastric Alkalinizers 18
Metronidazole 16
Miconazole 15
Sulfinpyrazone 16
Voriconazole 15
Glycopyrrolate
Donepezil 38
Galantamine 38
Rivastigmine 38
Goji. See Herbal
Interaction Chart
Grapefruit
Alfentanil 77
Alfuzosin 2
Almotriptan 100
Amiodarone 5
Amprenavir 26
Anxiolytics-Hypnotics
(CYP3A4 Substrates) 28
Aripiprazole 22
Atazanavir 26
Atorvastatin 55
Avanafil 80
Bedaquiline 97
Cabozantinib 61
Calcium channel blockers
33
Carbamazepine 35
Clozapine 22
Colchicine 42
Corticosteroids 45
Crizotinib 61
Cyclosporine 58
Daclatasvir 26
Darunavir 26
Dasatinib 61
Delavirdine 26
Disopyramide 5

140

141

142

143

144

145

146

148

150

151

152

153

155

156

159

HORN AND HANSTEN'S
DRUG INTERACTION PROBABILITY SCALE

The Drug Interaction Probability Scale (DIPS) is designed to assess the probability of a causal relationship between a drug interaction and an event.

Directions: Circle the appropriate answer for each question and sum the score. Use "Unknown or NA" if a) you do not have the information, or b) the question is not applicable.

---

1. Are there credible reports of this interaction in humans?
   Yes +1, No –1, Unknown or NA 0

2. Is the observed interaction consistent with the known interactive properties of the precipitant drug?   Yes +1, No –1, Unknown or NA 0

3. Is the observed interaction consistent with the known interactive properties of the object drug?   Yes +1, No –1, Unknown or NA 0

4. Is the event consistent with the known or reasonable time course of the interaction (onset and/or offset)?   Yes +1, No –1, Unknown or NA 0

5. Did the interaction remit upon dechallenge of the precipitant drug with no change in the object drug?   Yes +1, No –2, Unknown or NA 0

6. Did the interaction reappear when the precipitant drug was readministered with continued use of the object drug?   Yes +2, No –1, Unknown or NA 0

7. Are there reasonable alternative causes for the event?[a]
   Yes –1, No +1, Unknown or NA 0

8. Was the object drug detected in the blood or other fluids in concentrations consistent with the proposed interaction?   Yes +1, No 0, Unknown or NA 0

9. Was the drug interaction confirmed by any objective evidence consistent with the effects on the object drug (other than drug concentrations)?
   Yes +1, No 0, Unknown or NA 0

10. Was the reaction greater when the precipitant drug dose was increased or less when the precipitant drug dose was decreased?
    Yes +1, No –1, Unknown or NA 0

---

a. Consider clinical conditions, other drugs, lack of compliance, risk factors. A "NO" answer presumes that enough information was presented so that one would expect any alternative causes to be mentioned.

Total score_____	Highly Probable	>8
	Probable	5-8
	Possible	2-4
	Doubtful	<2

For more details see Horn JR, Hansten PD, Chan L-N. *Proposal for a New Tool to Evaluate Drug Interaction Cases*, Ann Pharmacotherapy 2007;41:674-680. The Drug Interaction Probability Scale is based on the Naranjo ADR Probability Scale adapted from Naranjo CA et al. Clin Pharmacol Ther 1981;30:239.

36123175R00105

Made in the USA
San Bernardino, CA
13 July 2016